THE CONFUSION ABOUT CHIROPRACTORS

**what they are, what they do,
and what they can do for you**

by
Dr. Richard E. DeRoeck

Impulse Publishing
Danbury, Connecticut

THE CONFUSION ABOUT CHIROPRACTORS
What They Are, What They Do, and What They Can Do For You

By
Dr. Richard E. DeRoeck

The information in this book is not intended as medical advice. Its intention is strictly educational. It is assumed that the reader will consult a health professional as needs dictate.

FIRST EDITION

Library of Congress Cataloging-in-Publication Data

DeRoeck, Richard E., 1946 -

The confusion about chiropractors.

    Includes Index.
    1. Chiropractic - Popular works.   2. Consumer education.
I. Title.
RZ244.D47   1989   615.5'34   88-34763
ISBN 0-923748-25-3

ACKNOWLEDGEMENTS

I wish to acknowledge my gratitude and indebtedness to the following people for the support and assistance they gave me during the preparation of this book, from the development of the manuscript all the way through to the finished product. At the risk of inevitably omitting some, the list includes:

Dr. Marino Passero for his critical insights and encouragement.

Joan Baldwin and Jacki Holterman, my office assistants, for their patience, understanding, encouragement, and supportive help in tending to the many details of manuscript preparation, and for tirelessly putting up with the ideas I ran by them.

My colleagues, Drs. Ed Markowitz and Richard Bailey, for providing the space for me to complete all the work necessary in the preparation of the book, and for their reliable encouragement.

Dr. Jack Chinsky, my friend, for always being there when the going got tough, and for believing in me.

Dan Poynter, for showing me the way to get it into print.

Jay Garon, for his tireless efforts in my behalf, and for his enthusiastic response to my ideas for this book.

All the people at Graphic Presentations, especially Patricia Montague, for their professional expertise and patient assistance during the design and typesetting phase of the project.

The many people at BookCrafters, especially Charlene Tanay, for their personal attention, caring, and the beautiful finished product.

And finally, Jacki Hanson-DeRoeck, my wife, not only for her loving support, encouragement and absolute belief in me every step of the way, but for her very skilled assistance in the design of the book and the Impulse Publishing logo.

Thank you all. Without your help, I have no idea how this book would have turned out.

Richard E. DeRoeck, D.C.

To Christian Richard DeRoeck, my greatest source of inspiration.

And to the memory of Dr. Joseph Janse, whose absolute dedication taught me the meaning of the word professionalism.

And to my patients, who continue to teach me daily.

ABOUT THE AUTHOR

Dr. Richard DeRoeck has been a practicing chiropractic physician since 1976, and is currently engaged in active practice in Danbury, Connecticut. His background and training in the health field began as a Health and Physical Education major at Queens College in New York City, from where he graduated with a Bachelor of Arts degree. He taught Health and Physical Education for several years, during which time he earned a Master of Science degree in Health from Herbert H. Lehman College, also in New York City. He attended the National College of Chiropractic in Lombard, Illinois from 1973 to 1976, and graduated Cum Laude with a Bachelor of Science in Human Biology as well as the Doctor of Chiropractic degree. He has been both a District Director and Journal Editor of the Connecticut Chiropractic Association, and is also a member of the American Chiropractic Association and the Greater Danbury Chiropractic Association. He has written numerous articles for chiropractic publications, and is now publishing books for the purpose of educating the public about Chiropractic, Health and Well-Being. He is committed to making a difference in the public perception and understanding of the Chiropractic profession, as well as in the degree to which people generally take responsibility for their well-being.

TABLE OF CONTENTS

FOREWORD

For the past 25 years, there has been a concerted effort on the part of Organized Medicine — spearheaded by the American Medical Association and eleven other "medical fraternities" — to suppress and eliminate the entire profession of Chiropractic.

Why? Why would the group be so antagonistic? Why would it hurl slurs about Chiropractic being an "unscientific cult," or try to denigrate the profession in the eyes of the American public by making it seem as if chiropractors were *uneducated opportunists*, or, even worse, try to deprive chiropractors of third-party insurance coverage and hospital privileges (as if these people owned and paid for the hospitals!)? Why have chiropractors been denied use of such facilities, denied referral privileges, and denied access to medical postgraduate courses?

Obviously, for Medicine to offer such a unified front against an entire healing profession means, from my perspective, that that profession offers an economic and philosophic threat. And, indeed it does.

Chiropractic is the second-largest healing profession and, potentially, the primary health profession of the future — especially as practiced by those chiropractors who do not merely adjust the body's vertebral subluxations, but who, rather, perceive and define "wellness" as a state of *balance* and *internal harmony,* and help their patients to strike such a balance. The chiropractor is uniquely suited to helping patients understand how balance and imbalance occur, and to intervening in a non-invasive and non-toxic manner to help bring back normal function.

In this particular book, Dr. DeRoeck has provided a sojourn into understanding Chiropractic from a *wholistic* perspective. It is a meaningful handbook for any person wanting to understand how to have an intelligent dialog with his or her chiropractor, and for anyone wishing to understand the chiropractor's orientation and perspective, specific to this healing art. The book is a useful tool, an important resource book, and a book that will certainly stand on its own among the finer books of its kind in the future.

Gary Null

Gary Null is a well-known and highly-regarded journalist in the area of natural, wholistic health care. He has written numerous books and articles on the subject, and is the host of a radio talk show in New York City.

INTRODUCTION: A Personal Perspective

Imagine yourself, for a moment, being a chiropractor. What do you suppose it would feel like? What kinds of thoughts would occupy your mind? What kind of knowledge would you possess? How do you imagine people would relate to you, and what would they think of you?

You can probably imagine yourself being practically anything else in the world: an actor, an entertainer, a professional athlete, a surgeon, an airline pilot, a newspaper reporter, an attorney, a police officer. With regard to each of these occupations, you are most likely able to fantasize about what it would feel like, how you would act, and how people would interact with you. You probably have some idea of what your work would be like, what kind of specialized training you would need, and what expertise you would need to have in each occupation.

I suspect, however, that it is difficult for you to imagine yourself being a chiropractor. It is probably safe to assume that you wouldn't even know where to begin.

What, after all, is a chiropractor, and what does he or she do? The majority of people in our society could not accurately answer those questions. Most people, in fact, don't know the first thing about the subject. You are in the majority if you have never been to a chiropractor, you don't know any chiropractors personally, and you have at best a foggy notion of what chiropractors do. Not only that, but it is very likely that you have read or heard some unflattering things about chiropractors, and so your impression is that they are fringe practitioners of some sort. It is doubtful that you have any knowledge of the kind of education chiropractors have, but you probably suspect that it is nowhere near the calibre of medical, dental, or veterinary education. You may not even think that a chiropractor must attend college to receive his or her training, or that there are any requirements for licensure as a chiropractor.

In contrast to the medical doctor, who is esteemed, the chiropractor is generally held in suspicion. Certainly, it is felt, chiropractors aren't *real* doctors. The chiropractor is somebody you may consider seeing if you want your back "cracked," whatever that is. Or, perhaps the chiropractor is somebody you wouldn't go to on a bet. If you're like most people, the very thought frightens you. Indeed, if you suspected that you had a serious problem of some kind, it's probably safe to say that you wouldn't consider visiting a chiropractor for treatment. Really now, what in the world could a *chiropractor* do for something serious?

If you are a person who has been to a chiropractor, this assessment still probably pertains to you. If you have been a chiropractic patient — even one who has obtained wondrous results — it's a safe bet that you don't know exactly what it is chiropractors do, or why it works. You probably have very little idea about what kinds of problems, other than the one you had, chiropractors can help. And you probably make a distinction between chiropractors and "regular" doctors.

All of this underscores my purpose in writing this book. People need to have a clear understanding of chiropractic health care. It's vital to the profession and to all the people who stand to benefit from chiropractic care - namely every man, woman and child walking on the planet.

Chiropractic (the name comes from the Greek, "to do by hand") happens to be a remarkably effective form of health care, but one that exists in almost total isolation from the rest of the health care system in our society. Whereas all of us have grown up with a deep-rooted inherent medical orientation, we — both laymen and health professionals alike — are essentially ignorant about chiropractic principles. What's worse, many people — and, especially physicians — *think* they have an accurate understanding about Chiropractic

14

but really don't, and are therefore propagating myth and misconception. Because of that, many people who could benefit tremendously from chiropractic care are frightened off.

You may be wondering how this could happen. If Chiropractic is so remarkable, why doesn't everybody know about it and how is it that not even the rest of the health care community is aware of its capabilities?

You will understand all of this and more after reading this book. My purpose is to set the record straight about Chiropractic, so that we no longer have a confused and uninformed (or worse, a *misinformed*) public.

I think you will enjoy THE CONFUSION ABOUT CHIROPRACTORS. I have endeavored to make it informative and yet entertaining, and have studiously avoided making you plod knee-deep through scientific jargon.

Hopefully, this book will accomplish two objectives. First, it will educate you about Chiropractic in a way that enables you to understand its principles, realize and appreciate its value, know where it fits into our system of health care, and overcome any apprehensions you may have about seeking chiropractic care. And secondly, it will give you a look at just what it's like to swim against the current as a chiropractor, dealing with the myths, misconceptions, attitudes and fears of a confused public.

I truly hope this book makes a difference for you. If so, please recommend it to friends. It's time to end the confusion about chiropractors.

Richard E. DeRoeck, D.C.

1

Why Would Anyone Want to be a Chiropractor?

Sometimes they're subtle about it. They'll ask a sincere question like, "What made you decide to become a chiropractor?" Implicit in that question is another: *"Why would anyone want to be a chiropractor?"*

Sometimes they're not so subtle: "Why didn't you look into becoming a *regular* doctor?"

Once in a while, they get right to the point: "Didn't you ever want to be a *real* doctor?"

Patients, friends, casual acquaintances alike are prone to asking the question. It's less a question, really, than a reflection of the popular conception that chiropractors are inferior, second-rate practitioners.

The fact of the matter is that people who ask these questions don't mean anything personal by them. They are simply reacting to their remote impression of what chiropractors are. It is rarely a product of direct personal experience, but is usually the result of something they either read or heard, often from a source that also did not get it firsthand.

It is interesting to observe the way people react when they are casually introduced to a chiropractor in a social situation. One very common reaction is the rather patronizing remark "Oh, a chiropractor! My father (mother, brother, etc.) swears by his chiropractor." Even though it is meant as a gesture of approval, it has a hollow ring to it.

Another common statement is, "My sister (brother, mother, father, boss, etc.) really *believes* in you people." This seems to place chiropractors right up there with such luminaries as Santa Claus, the Easter Bunny, and the Tooth Fairy — creatures that exist only in the mind of the believer.

Such comments might appear harmless, but they underscore the underlying issue here, which is whether or not chiropractors are doctors, worthy of the same stature as other doctors. The unequivocal answer is *yes*.

The following story describes how this author decided to become a chiropractor.

I used to be a high school health education teacher. For a number of reasons, I did not find it totally fulfilling, and I made the decision to find a different profession before too much more time passed by. As I began investigating the possibilities, the only thing I was sure of was that I wanted to remain in a health-related field. It was consistent with my background and training, and had always held great interest for me.

During my search for a new career, the field of Chiropractic came up from time to time. I knew absolutely nothing about the profession; I had never been to a chiropractor, and had scarcely heard of them, much less know what they did. The closest I had ever come to experiencing Chiropractic was vicariously, through a few treatments that my brother had received for a back problem, along with having heard my father talk about a chiropractor he knew casually who, he said, seemed "well off." But I had never really given the profession much thought. One day, while having lunch in the faculty cafeteria, I struck up a conversation with an industrial arts teacher whom I will call Frank. I mentioned that I was looking to change professions, and was curious about this field known as Chiropractic. That's all I had to say.

Frank proceeded to tell me about an experience that had changed his life, and was — unbeknownst to me — about to change mine.

About two years earlier, Frank had been involved in a serious automobile accident that had left him paralyzed below the waist. Following the accident, he had had absolutely no use of his legs.

After many grueling months of healing and rehabilitation, he was told by several of "the best neurosurgeons in New York" that he would be a paraplegic for the remainder of his life. Frank, a vital and active man, was devastated.

Totally out of desperation, Frank's brother, Bob, suggested that Frank see Bob's chiropractor. Feeling that he certainly had nothing to lose, Frank agreed.

After examining Frank, the chiropractor then made what I still consider to be a very foolish statement. "Frank," he said, "If you had come to see me right after the accident, I could have had you walking right away. As it is, though, it will take me about two months." Considering the circumstances, Frank figured he could probably live with the two-month wait. The chiropractor's statement might have sounded like the empty promise of a huckster taking advantage of a man's desperation, especially in light of the prognosis Frank had received from the neurosurgeons. Certainly, that's what it would have sounded like to me, except for one notable detail: two months later, almost to the day, Frank was walking. Not only was he walking, but he was soon back to playing golf and tennis, and doing whatever else he wished. He was completely cured.

The reaction of the neurosurgeons was predictable. They said, "It was one of those freak things — a coincidence. It would no doubt have happened on its own, without the intervention of the chiropractor. He's just lucky the chiropractor didn't really hurt him, or do anything to interfere with his miraculous response."

On the basis of Frank's experience, I decided to look more seriously into Chiropractic, and I ultimately decided to enter the profession.

Frank's story is no fluke. Others like it occur almost daily in chiropractors' offices all over the world. A large percentage, perhaps the majority, of chiropractors originally enter the profession because of similar experiences of their own or of people close to them.

Chiropractors are doctors, make no mistake about it. The terms "chiropractor" and "chiropractic physician" are interchangeable according to state statutes. Upon graduation from chiropractic college, the degree *Doctor of Chiropractic* is conferred, an advanced professional degree recognized by the U.S. Office of Education.

Chiropractors are not medical doctors, but then again, neither are dentists (Doctor of Dental Science), podiatrists (Doctor of Podiatric Medicine), osteopaths (Doctor of Osteopathy), or optometrists (Optometric Doctor). You don't have to be a medical doctor to be a doctor. People just think you do.

Chiropractors are licensed in every state and, with few exceptions, are acknowledged by the various states as *primary physicians*, along with allopaths (MD's) and osteopaths. A primary physician is one who is qualified, by virtue of his or her training, to serve as a "portal of entry" into the health care system — a doctor to whom you may go confidently with virtually any health problem, and who is trained to diagnose your condition and either treat you or refer you to another physician better suited to render care for that particular condition. The fact that chiropractors are licensed and recognized as primary physicians by the state licensing boards around the country — especially in consideration of all the opposition the profession has encountered — demonstrates that these state agencies are satisfied that chiropractors are totally capable and worthy of that responsibility.

In order to be granted a license to practice Chiropractic, one must (a) be a graduate of an accredited chiropractic college, and (b) pass a licensing examination administered by the Board of Chiropractic Examiners in the state in which the doctor wishes to practice. In some states, this Board is made up solely of other chiropractors, while in others the Board includes both medical doctors and lay persons. Regardless of its makeup, the Board of Chiropractic Examiners is under the auspices of the State Department of Health. The licensing examination typically consists of both written and practical segments that allow the Board to accurately assess an applicant's competence. In addition, many states also require successful completion of a very thorough examination given by the National Board of Chiropractic Examiners. This test may be taken by a chiropractic student during his or her final year of school. The licensure requirements to practice Chiropractic are strict and rigid, and anyone who obtains a license to practice Chiropractic has indeed earned the right to be called "Doctor."

This discussion highlights three important points. First, chiropractors are doctors. Second, chiropractors are not medical doctors. And third, medical doctors are not the only people entitled to the appellation "Doctor." Anyone who has been granted an advanced professional degree by an accredited degree-granting institution is equally deserving of that privilege.

The following story typifies how little people know about Chiropractic, and the way in which the profession and its practitioners are perceived by a large segment of the population.

When I was preparing to go away to chiropractic college, a few close friends threw a party for me. I was, of course, very touched by the gesture — until I quickly discovered that whatever levity there was to be that evening would be at my expense.

The highlight of the evening occurred when two of the men, who had quietly left the room earlier, re-entered dressed as *witch doctors*, complete with masks, bizarre necklaces, spears, and body paint. They proceeded to perform their unique interpretation of a chiropractic ceremonial dance.

After they finished, they presented me with all the regalia they had used, along with a scrapbook they had painstakingly made for me. It contained a number of unusual cartoons and photographs taken from newspapers and magazines — two-headed creatures, witch doctors, *Guinness Book* oddballs - each accompanied by an appropriately comical chiropractic caption. Many hours of work had obviously gone into this most humiliating experience, and I had to remind myself that these were good friends, who were on my side!

Certainly, that parody was meant in fun, but the whole scenario exemplifies a common perception of Chiropractic.

2 Chiropractic Education

When I opened my first chiropractic practice in 1977, I wasn't terribly busy at first, a condition not uncommon among new practitioners. As a result, to this day I have a fairly vivid recollection of nearly every one of my patients from that period.

Another thing that I recall is that — also not unlike other new practitioners — I was not secure enough in my new role as a physician to just act naturally, and so I was prone to performing my "doctor act" and to being quite defensive about my credentials.

One patient I will probably never forget was a woman whom I will call Rose. Rose came to my office one day to become a new patient and, after filling out the necessary forms, was waiting in my office for me to enter to conduct the initial interview. (It had not taken me long, by the way, to discover that by making a patient wait for a few minutes, I could give the person the impression of being busy.)

On the wall behind my desk, I proudly displayed all my diplomas. Having the patient wait offered the additional advantage of allowing that person the opportunity to see those plaques and realize the superior nature and extent of my education.

When I entered the room. Rose was attentively studying my wall. She saw my two Bachelor's degrees, a Master's, and the Doctor of Chiropractic diploma. Noticing Rose's apparent interest in them, I rather smugly introduced myself: "Hello, I'm Doctor DeRoeck." Rose's matter-of-fact response left me speechless: "I didn't even know you went to college!"

That story illustrates a common misconception about chiropractic education. It seems that most people think our training must be quite meager — certainly, no match for medical education — and I don't doubt at all that there are some who think that a person could sign up for the course of study by filling out the inside of a matchbook cover.

The truth is far-removed from that notion. Chiropractic education begins with the prerequisite two years of pre-professional college study, with a concentration in human sciences. Although this two-year preliminary program is all that is required, the majority of entering chiropractic students possess at least a Bachelor's degree. Following the preliminary program, the aspirant then begins the Doctor of Chiropractic (DC) course of study at a chiropractic college accredited by the Commission on Accreditation of the Council on Chiropractic Education, which is in turn approved by the United States Office of Education.

The DC program consists of five academic years of study, usually divided into ten trimesters or semesters. During the first five trimesters, the student chiropractor studies the *basic sciences* in a curriculum much like those studied in medical, dental, or veterinary schools. Included among the subjects studied intensively are: organic chemistry, biochemistry, anatomy of the musculoskeletal system (including limbs, trunk and head), anatomy of the internal structures of the body (including all of the organs, blood vessels and internal systems), neuroanatomy (the anatomy of the brain, spinal cord, and entire nervous system), physiology (how all those systems function), neurophysiology, pathology (the study of disease), bacteriology, histology (the microscopic study of body tissues), and microbiology.

The second five trimesters are devoted to the concentrated study of the *clinical sciences,* including: X-ray physics, X-ray positioning, X-ray interpretation, laboratory diagnosis (blood and urine studies), physical examination and diagnosis, neurology, orthopedics, cardiology, obstetrics and gynecology, pediatrics, geriatrics, dermatology, GI/GU, physical therapy, nutrition, and chiropractic treatment techniques.

During the final year of his or her study, the student chiropractor sees patients in a college-affiliated clinic, where the *externship* program prepares the graduating chiropractor in patient care and practice management.

In addition to this basic chiropractic curriculum, there are *residencies* available in both radiology and orthopedics. A chiropractic graduate may apply to study an additional three years in order to become either a chiropractic radiologist or a chiropractic orthopedist. The training received in these programs is highly specialized, and both of these chiropractic specialists are the equal of their medical counterparts in terms of diagnostic acumen.

The primary difference between chiropractic and medical education is in the emphasis of the coursework and preparation. The medical curriculum, of course, is designed to prepare the medical student to diagnose and combat systemic diseases, with great emphasis on the use of drugs and surgery. The chiropractic curriculum, on the other hand, is designed to prepare the chiropractic student to evaluate and conservatively manage conditions from a *holistic* (or, "wholistic") point of view, in which the various factors that affect a person's health are taken into consideration, including such factors as diet, nutritional supplementation, exercise, stress, and lifestyle.

In the chiropractic curriculum, great emphasis is placed on the functional dynamics (mechanics) of the body, and especially the dynamics of *the spine.* The human spine is studied intensively with regard to its structure, function, and relationship to overall body function, the end result being that the chiropractor has no equal when it comes to understanding the spine and its various disorders, or the conservative treatment and management of spinal conditions. The spine is intimately related to both body mechanics and the functional control the nervous system exerts over the entire body, and is frequently involved in disorders of both (see Chapter Five).

Can we say that chiropractic education is comparable to medical, osteopathic and dental education as far as qualification for clinical practice is concerned? Yes, absolutely. The chiropractic physician has been well-schooled in the basic sciences and is thoroughly trained in the clinical and diagnostic sciences, just like his or her counterparts in the other health professions. The fact of the matter is that the chiropractic curriculum actually consists of *more* classroom hours of basic and clinical science study than the medical equivalent.

From a personal point of view, speaking as someone who has experienced his share of college and graduate study, I found my experience in chiropractic college to be, by far, the most rigorous and challenging test of my intellectual and scholastic ability. The most brilliant, knowledgeable, and academically accomplished people I have ever known are former chiropractic classmates of mine who are now practicing chiropractic physicians. The chiropractor can hold his or her head up high when in the spotlight of academia.

One of the reasons for the many misconceptions about the quality of chiropractic education is the abundance of anti-Chiropractic propaganda that, for years, has flatly proclaimed that chiropractors are unscientific and untrained to diagnose and treat human disease. That assertion is totally untrue today, but is, to some extent, a case of pointing a finger at what once may have been and proclaiming it as existing in the present.

Chiropractic began as an organized profession in 1895, when its founder, a self-styled healer named Daniel David Palmer, purportedly restored the hearing of a man who had fallen deaf by performing a mobilizing treatment of the man's spine (see Chapter Five). The early educational program organized by Palmer was admittedly crude, abbreviated and inadequate.

Over the years, however, the profession has elevated its educational standards to the current level, which is beyond reproach. Today, chiropractic colleges are sanctioned as degree-granting institutions by the same regional accrediting agencies that regulate all other colleges and universities. If the educational curriculum of such a facility is not of superior quality, or if the qualifications and credentials of its faculty are inadequate, the school will not receive accreditation. If accreditation is granted, it is earned.

Organized Medicine — the source of the anti-Chiropractic propaganda — appears to demonstrate a conveniently short memory. As recently as 1910, medical education was regarded as "disgraceful and shameful." A renowned educator named Dr. Abraham Flexner was retained by the Carnegie Foundation to make a study of existing medical schools at that time, and his resulting report, *Medical Education in the United States and Canada*, concluded that most of the 155 medical schools were merely fly-by-night diploma mills that extracted tuition from unqualified students, offered inferior medical courses and issued medical degrees. Just as the quality of medical education has had to be dramatically upgraded since the Flexner Report, so, too, has chiropractic education been similarly upgraded since its inception.

If there is any one area in which chiropractic education falls short, it would have to be the lack of opportunity to personally experience seeing patients with health problems covering the entire spectrum. Chiropractic training is limited to college-affiliated clinics. No part of it takes place in hospitals or other medical facilities. As a result, the chiropractic student has a limited opportunity to develop the keen diagnostic acumen that comes from seeing all the various conditions in real life. Although the student chiropractor has a textbook knowledge of the entire range of human health problems, his or her experience is generally limited to those considered *musculoskeletal* in nature. The outcome is that the practicing chiropractor must be especially alert for indications of systemic problems in every patient, although he or she has never actually witnessed many of them.

Medical critics of Chiropractic are fast to point out that shortcoming, but loath to acknowledge that it is the medical community that has denied chiropractic students access to this all-important arena of training. Up to this point in time, chiropractors have generally been prevented from gaining hospital privileges or from taking advantage of their fertile training ground.

31

Although it has been my experience that the vast majority of chiropractors develop an outstanding degree of diagnostic expertise, there is no question that the firsthand experience lacking in chiropractic training would hasten and enhance the process. What is obviously needed is a greater spirit of cooperation between the medical and chiropractic professions, which would benefit all concerned.

POSTGRADUATE EDUCATION

The chiropractor's education doesn't end with graduation from chiropractic college. In a very real sense, it is only the beginning. There are innumerable programs in postgraduate education for the practicing chiropractor. Not only are seminars and workshops available on a perpetual basis, but it is absolutely essential for any doctor in the field to be continually involved in postgraduate courses if he or she is to stay current.

There are programs available in virtually every chiropractic specialty, as well as in the diagnosis and management of soft tissue injuries, disc syndromes, and other common and difficult conditions. Practically every accredited chiropractic college sponsors such postgraduate education, which is made available all over the United States.

The colleges also offer comprehensive 360-hour programs of study in orthopedics, neurology, radiology, and sports medicine. Upon successful completion of each of these programs, a doctor is qualified to sit for an examination to be awarded Diplomate status by Chiropractic Boards in the corresponding specialties.

In addition to those programs of study, which are purely Chiropractic-oriented, there are numerous seminars and conferences that are interdisciplinary in nature, on such topics as low back pain, nutrition, fitness, biochemical imbalances, and virtually every other area of common interest. At these conferences, physicians from every discipline have the opportunity to exchange views and perspectives.

Chiropractic education is anything but deficient. It is thorough, comprehensive, ongoing and highly technical, and matches up well against any educational program in any professional or technical discipline.

3
We Don't Get No Respect

WE DON'T GET NO RESPECT

Comedian Rodney Dangerfield has built an entire career out of his "I don't get no respect" routine. I think it's safe to say that Mr. Dangerfield places a very distant second behind the Chiropractic profession in the "no respect" department.

Relatively few people — other than chiropractors themselves — know exactly what chiropractors do. That includes members of the general population as well as members of the health care community. Chiropractors treat from 7 to 10 percent of the American population, which is about twice what it was in 1980. That leaves approximately 90% of the American people who don't have the foggiest notion about what chiropractors do. What's more, even our own patients — the 7-10% of the population that we *do* treat — have *only* the foggiest notion.

This, of course, is a gross generalization; there are some exceptions to this picture. But, by and large, Chiropractic is the best-kept secret in health care.

There are many reasons for this, which you will discover as you read on. But the primary reason that so few people know what chiropractors do is that Chiropractic is just not a part of the mainstream of healthcare. The mainstream is very much the domain of the medical profession. Yes, it's true that over the years — usually in spite of medical opposition — other professions have slipped through the cracks into the system. But make no mistake about it: the health care system in our society remains a monarchy, and the medical profession reigns supreme.

It is no secret that the medical profession has always been generally opposed to Chiropractic. To confirm this, all one would have to do is ask anyone who has ever told his or her medical doctor about having been to a chiropractor. Typical responses range from very mild ("Well, go if you want, but it won't do you any good") to the more severe ("What?!!! Don't you know that those people can *hurt* you?").

Political Medicine (i.e., the American Medical Association) has always gone to great lengths to influence public opinion, legislation, and even its own membership against Chiropractic. As a result, medical doctors tend to regard us as charlatans, the general public has a decidedly negative impression of Chiropractic, and probably our own mothers hold us in suspicion. It's not a pretty picture.

To add insult to injury, the Chiropractic profession hasn't done very much in its own behalf to sway public opinion in its favor. In earlier times, chiropractors frequently made extravagant claims about the health benefits of Chiropractic, touting it as the cure for everything from acne to cancer to the plague. Lacking evidence to support such claims, they were not particularly well received by the scientific community. The chiropractors undoubtedly made the assertions they did to attract attention to themselves, since Chiropractic was light years from mainstream health care at that time. While the claims were exaggerated and ill-conceived, they did *not* indicate — as detractors proclaimed — that Chiropractic was of no value whatsoever. Both positions were unfounded. However, it's safe to say that the zealots did little to further their own cause, and much to fuel a fire that has burned for years in the medical community.

Today, Organized Chiropractic appears to have taken the diametrically opposed tack. The Chiropractic stance today is one of *quiet effectiveness*. We chiropractors quietly go about the business of achieving remarkable results in patient care, and *nobody knows about it.* We have developed, and we continue to refine, an art and a science that is far and away the best treatment for some of the most common and troublesome ailments, *and nobody knows about it.* We have a discipline that just may be able to prevent disease and prolong life better than anything else can, *and nobody knows about it.* If everyone knew what *we* know about Chiropractic, people would be literally breaking down our doors to get what we have to offer. There wouldn't be nearly enough chiropractic offices to hold all the patients wanting care. Instead, though, the chiropractor toils in relative anonymity.

There are, however, a large number of chiropractors who have very busy offices. As in any profession, the combination of competent care, quality service, good results and friendly patient relations works to generate referrals into the chiropractor's office. The problem, though, is that the chiropractor has a perpetual uphill struggle to prove himself or herself to a wary public. Many patients only visit the chiropractor out of desperation, after nothing else has worked for them. Some even mention their skepticism, practically daring the doctor to help them.

As a result, a climate has developed in which some chiropractors feel the need to resort to competitive advertising. This "Eat at Joe's" mentality does little to elevate the image of the profession, but the doctors who are involved in it feel it is necessary for survival. Competitiveness, rather than cooperation, is fostered by these circumstances. Many times, as soon as there are a handful of chiropractors in a geographical area, some begin to complain of "too much competition." Unfortunately, in one sense they are right: chiropractors are all in competition for the same tiny piece of the health care market. The Chiropractic profession desperately needs to begin educating the public about what it is chiropractors actually do. There are more than enough people out there who could benefit from chiropractic care, but most of them don't know it. It is the job of the Chiropractic profession to tell them.

INTERPROFESSIONAL RELATIONS

Even though many chiropractors have friends and relatives who are members of the medical and legal professions, those professions generally show little regard for Chiropractic. This fact has little to do with the personal credibility of the individual chiropractors. What it involves is the credibility of the *image* of Chiropractic. There are medical doctors who won't even take a telephone call from a chiropractor inquiring about a patient. Attorneys and judges typically place little credence in courtroom testimony provided by chiropractors.

In a courtroom, the orthopedic surgeon is generally regarded as a much more reliable and credible expert witness than the chiropractor. This is true in spite of the fact that the chiropractor understands joint function and joint and soft tissue injury and disability as well as or better than the orthopedist. Many attorneys studiously avoid having chiropractors testify for their clients — and will often advise a client to discontinue chiropractic care — because they and the judges have doubts about the validity of Chiropractic and about the chiropractor's expertise. Here again, it is not that these people have taken the time to learn about Chiropractic or the nature of the chiropractor's training. It's just that they have acquired the prevailing prejudice against Chiropractic. So, with judge, jury and attorney (even the one in whose favor the chiropractor testifies) all convinced of Chiropractic inferiority, one can easily see why the chiropractor is frequently disregarded as both the treating physician and expert witness.

The issue of Chiropractic's negative image and lack of respect is one whose roots are deep, strong, and well-established. In the chapters to follow, the source of the problem will be examined, as will the facts about Chiropractic, so that myth and misconception can be separated from fact.

4
Who Died and Left Them Boss?

In order to put the issues at hand into perspective, we must take a philosophical look at the nature of the health care system in our society, and at some of the beliefs which we have formed about it. Only by uprooting these beliefs can we make room for a new and more accurate point of view.

During the evolution of our system of health care, certain beliefs have become accepted as fundamental truths. Certain points of view have become accepted as *the only* points of view, never questioned or challenged. This kind of rigidity is always a deterrent to growth and progress wherever it occurs, and this is certainly the case with regard to our health care system.

MEDICAL SUPREMACY

First of all, our culture has long accepted the premise that "health care" means "medical care." As far as most people are concerned, there is no other form of health care than medical care. There is a cultural notion that the medical profession boasts the only people who are suitably trained and prepared to care for our health. The medical doctor is widely regarded as the caretaker of our health.

From birth, all of us receive a carefully-ingrained medical orientation. It is the medical doctor who delivers us at birth, and the ceremony takes place in the medical temple, the hospital. It is the medical doctor whom we turn to when we become ill.

As we grow up, we learn to "go to the doctor" whenever we "come down with" an illness. As children, we read books such as, *A Visit to the Doctor*, and *Franny Goes to the Hospital* , which firmly establish in our minds the role of the medical doctor as the guardian of health.

Television shows and movies about doctors such as *Marcus Welby* and *Dr. Kildare* portray the MD as a hero, helping to position him in our eyes as the Supreme Being of health and health care. (There are some people, in fact, — doctors and patients alike — who seem to think that "MD" stands for "Medical Deity.")

The result of all of this conditioning is that we have developed an absolute, blind faith in the ability of "the doctor" to *fix* whatever goes wrong with us. Having such faith frees us from the concern and responsibility of caring for our own health.

OUR INTERPRETATION OF HEALTH

We have been trained to believe that "good health" is synonymous with "feeling good." As long as we aren't experiencing troublesome symptoms, we can consider ourselves to be in good health. We have been taught that we can just go about the business of living our lives, and as long as we feel alright, we're doing just fine. Certainly, we consider it perfectly *normal* to occasionally feel somewhat "under the weather," with a headache, a cold, the flu, or any of the array of so-called "normal" aches and pains. We know from experience that these problems will pass — although we may ultimately have to take some medication for them — and that normal health includes any and all of them. It is only when symptoms become significant enough to interfere with our lives that our health becomes a concern, and what we do when that happens is to "go to the doctor" for a *cure*.

HEALTH CARE

And then, when we go to the doctor, what is it that is done for us? After a brief examination, we are usually given a prescription for one medication or another for the purpose of relieving our symptoms. We are usually able to leave the doctor's office confident that we are not going to die and that the medication will have us feeling better before too long. And we know that if, for whatever reason, the medication doesn't work, there is always another to replace it. Moreover, we know that if the problem still doesn't respond after a number of medications have been tried, there is probably a surgical procedure that, although we may not be anxious to undergo it, can effect a cure. In any event, we know in our hearts that we have a health care system we can almost always count on to take care of our problems and keep us going. As far as most people are concerned, this is exactly the way health care should be.

MEDICAL TECHNOLOGY

As a society, we have developed a fascination for all the wondrous advances being made in medical technology. We now have surgical procedures that can restore detached limbs, transplant hearts, and even implant artificial ones. We can bypass clogged and diseased arteries and even transplant healthy ones in their place.

Billions of dollars are devoted to the research and development of these and other advances, in order that we can come up with ways of combatting the various diseases that plague our culture so that we can prolong life. Every year, dozens upon dozens of new drugs are placed on the market to help give us greater relief from all of our various symptoms. As a result of all these technological advances, we have seen the average lifespan extended to approximately 75 years.

THE CAUSE OF DISEASE

We all know, of course, that germs cause disease. More specifically, although many diseases aren't caused by germs, the "germ theory" of disease is widely accepted in our culture with no question.

Those conditions that are not germ-induced — like headache, backache, fatigue, depression, heart disease, stroke, ulcers, and cancer — seem to just "attack" us for no apparent reason. Excluding these ailments, however, most of us are satisfied that the germ theory accounts for the cause of a vast array of diseases.

A CLOSER LOOK AT THESE BELIEFS

About Medical Supremacy: Where is it written that medical doctors are the only ones qualified to care for patients? Who says that the medical system is the only system — or even the best system, for that matter — available to us for our health care needs? Think about it — who says so?

They do, that's who. The medical profession has very effectively established itself as the guardian of our health, unwilling to share that responsibility with anyone else. Somewhere along the line, medical doctors established themselves as the only *real* doctors, and *health care* became synonymous with *medical care.* It is almost a sacrilege to suggest otherwise. The medical approach to health and disease has come to be regarded as the only valid approach, with all others being suspect.

The fact is, there are a number of professionals who are every bit as qualified as the MD to care for our health. The podiatrist, the optometrist, the dentist, and the osteopath all are, as is the chiropractor. Medical doctors don't have a corner on the market of knowledge and expertise about health and disease, although they would have you think otherwise.

The customary medical approach is not always the best approach to health care. This is certainly true for a wide variety of our most common health problems, including most causes of headache, back pain, pain or numbness in the arms or legs, and many others. The fact of the matter is that by the time it really becomes necessary to employ the medical approach in the treatment of these problems, it is usually because other, more sensible approaches have been overlooked.

About Health: The previous statement is true because our cultural interpretation of health — which we have inherited from our health care system — is erroneous. We have been conditioned to believe that good health means simply having no symptoms, and that we're healthy as long as we feel well. This notion is disproven every day, every time a person suddenly drops dead when in apparent good health. According to the common perception, you can be perfectly healthy one minute, and perfectly dead the next. It just doesn't happen that way.

Good health is much more than the mere absence of symptoms. Good health means that your level of well-being is far above that at which problems exist and symptoms develop. A healthy heart, for instance, will not just suddenly stop working. A heart that fails has been gradually deteriorating as the result of a disease process, a process that often develops silently, with no symptoms.

Good health is a level far above "normal" health. It exists in an arena that extends a great distance, in fact, above what we consider "normal." (Figure 1).

Rather than being defined merely by the absence of symptoms, the upper limit of what's available to us in the area of well-being is what can be called "Optimal Health." This can be defined as that level of wellness at which every tissue, cell and organ in one's body is functioning optimally. While probably just hypothetical — there is no level of health at which one could still not improve — it is approachable, and it is a status far superior to the mere absence of symptoms. But it cannot be attained within the context of the symptom/relief mentality of our medical system. Optimal health is a *journey*, not a destination, and it must be undertaken with purposeful, diligent effort rather than the random monitoring of symptoms.

THE CONFUSION ABOUT CHIROPRACTORS

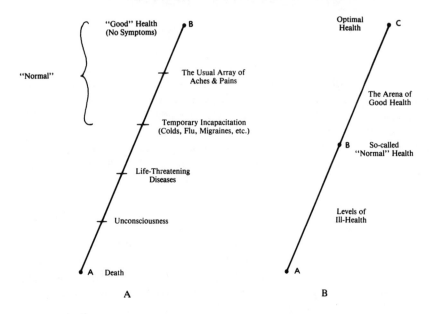

Figure 1. A, The typical interpretation of health, with "No Symptoms" representing the highest level attainable. Notice that "Normal" health includes a variety of common ailments. B, The real continuum of health, extending upward beyond "Normal" health, towards Optimal Health.

About Health Care: Because of our society's orientation toward health, we exist in a unique situation in which "health care" really isn't health care at all. It is more accurately described as *disease care,* or *crisis medicine.* In this system, as long as we don't suffer from any symptoms, we need pay no attention to our health, and the doctor has no real interest in seeing us. It is only after symptoms develop that our health becomes a concern, to us and to the doctor.

This approach to health care is an invalid one that serves us poorly. Since health is really a continuum that encompasses *all* levels of well-being, and a developing disease is not necessarily accompanied by symptoms, health care should be a matter of positive health promotion rather than crisis intervention.

It *is* true that medical groups and hospitals are now promoting programs that deal more in prevention, but don't let that mislead you. They are doing it for one reason, and one reason only: *because it's popular.* People have begun more and more to involve themselves in programs that help to promote good

48

health. The medical community recognizes this fact and is anxious to corner that portion of the health care market as well. But make no mistake about it, crisis care is still the cornerstone of the health care system.

The use of drugs to relieve our symptoms is a typical example of the shortsightedness of the medical approach. When symptoms appear — indicating a well-developed destructive process — medication is offered to *mask the symptoms*, so that we can go on with our lives. In essence, the fire rages on, but the alarm has been turned off. The disease process actually continues to develop and undermine the patient's health, and it does so with medical encouragement.

That is not to imply that drugs are never necessary, or that chiropractors do not believe in them. On the contrary. There are numerous instances in which medication is absolutely necessary, and medical technology is to be applauded for having developed the extremely effective preparations that are available for just such occasions.

What is wrong, however, is the "cart-before-the-horse" medical approach that emphasizes symptomatic care as its primary thrust. To administer a drug as a "cure" for a condition is to imply that the cause of the condition was that the patient's body lacked the drug to begin with. Except in rare cases — such as the administration of insulin to a diabetic (which actually doesn't address the question of *why* the person's pancreas quit producing insulin) — this is never true. Obviously, crisis medicine should always be available as an integral part of our health care system. But it, and the doctors who render such care, should comprise the *back line* of defense against disease. The front line should be devoted to *preventing* the cause of disease in the first place.

Medical technology, while it must continue to develop such crisis remedies as limb and organ replacement, needs to devote far more resources to prevention. We applaud ourselves for having extended our life expectancy to 75 years, when we should really be looking at why most of us don't live a normal, active, healthy lifetime of 100 years or more, which is our birthright. Instead of *expecting* to be weak, frail, arthritic, and debilitated by cancer or heart disease by age 70 — as we've been taught to do — we should have a health care system that empowers us to *really* reach old age, and to reach it with gusto. That is what health care should be about.

About the Cause of Disease: We have been taught to believe that germs cause disease. It's common knowledge, isn't it?

Sure it is, except for one thing: it isn't true. The idea that germs cause disease is not a fact at all. It's a *theory*, one of many on the subject of disease causation.

If germs caused diseases, anyone exposed to an organism that "caused" a particular disease would develop the condition. That isn't the way it happens. Bob and Betty could be in a room with someone suffering from pneumonia, and Bob might come down with the condition while Betty might not. In fact, if the germ theory were valid, we would all be sick most of the time. You see, we harbor in our digestive and respiratory tracts numerous organisms that are associated with a variety of diseases. But we generally never develop the conditions. Why not? Because *it's not the germ that causes the disease.*

Germs are *associated* with specific diseases. They must be present in order for the conditions to develop, but their mere presence doesn't necessarily lead to the disease process. The germ is only one of several factors that determine disease causation. It may, indeed, be the most important factor, since you could say that eliminating the germ eliminates the disease, but it is still only one of many factors. Other factors play a strong role in the disease process, regardless of whether or not micro-organisms are involved with the particular condition at all.

Generally speaking, the way these factors come into play is by affecting what is known as *tissue resistance*. Tissue resistance can be defined as *the ability of a person's body tissues to remain fully functional and healthy in the face of the presence of various disease-producing factors*. The degree to which your body tissues are able to resist the destructive effects of such factors is the degree to which you can resist disease. Inasmuch as the germs are more or less omnipresent, it would seem to make a great deal more sense to address those other health factors — which can be more easily controlled — than to wait until a disease develops and attack the "responsible" organism with drug therapy.

Among the factors that affect tissue resistance, thereby also influencing disease causation, are: *nutrition, exercise, stress, habits,* and *structural integrity* (the functional dynamics of the body). Largely ignored by the rest of the health care system, these factors are vitally important to health, and just happen to be the emphasis of Chiropractic health care. The chiropractor pays close attention to the way in which these factors are influencing the patient's well-being, and works with the patient to create the most favorable interplay of the various health factors.

By far, though, the most characteristic aspect of Chiropractic is its careful attention to the functional dynamics of *the spine*, and it is that focus that sets it apart.

5

The Spine: Lifeline of the Body

In all disease
Look first to the spine.

Hippocrates
The "Father of Medicine"

Like the well-known clothing store advertisement says, "An educated consumer is our best customer." Experience has shown that a person who fully understands and appreciates the fundamental principles and benefits of chiropractic care is more than likely to take advantage of those benefits by seeking care.

Chiropractic is truly unique among the healing arts. It deals with all the factors that influence health, but its principal focus is on just one: the structural dynamics of the body. More specifically even than that, Chiropractic addresses itself to the structural and functional dynamics of *the spine*, as it relates to the function of the body as a whole.

In order to fully understand Chiropractic and how it works, it is first necessary to understand the spine and the role it plays in overall body function.

THE NERVOUS SYSTEM

The human body is a remarkable structure of intricate simplicity. All of its complex biochemical reactions, all the activities of some 100 trillion cells and dozens of interdependent organs, are under the complete control of a single coordinating system. The *nervous system* — consisting of the brain, a dozen pairs of cranial nerves (nerves that originate in the head), the spinal cord, 31 pairs of spinal nerves that leave the spinal cord and form a network of offshoots like branches of a tree, and a handful of assorted specialty structures — generates and regulates all of the body's activities. Nothing occurs within the body without being caused or monitored by the nervous system.

The rather uncomplicated gross anatomy of the nervous system belies its complexity. Nobody knows exactly how the nervous system functions. We've been able to decipher many things about its function that have allowed us to understand its general patterns, but precisely how it works is another story. It remains a mystery that may never be unravelled.

For example, we know that the signals, or *impulses*, that travel throughout the nervous system resemble those of an electric current, but their exact nature is unknown. No one knows for certain how we are able to record and remember information, or think abstractly or creatively. We only know that we can. We can observe the channels of communication within the nervous system, but haven't the vaguest notion how it all happens.

Nevertheless, we know that the nervous system controls all bodily functions. Signals pass through the nervous system by the millions, conveying information back and forth between the brain and the rest of the body. Any interference with the transmission of any of these signals will necessarily interfere with the normal function of the body parts served by the signals.

Figure 2 depicts the major components of the human nervous system.

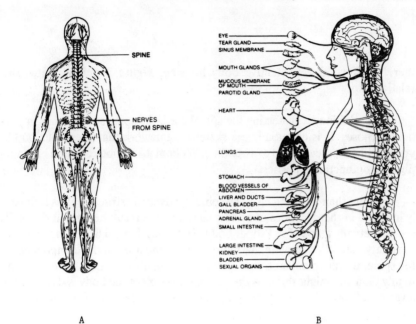

Figure 2. A, The Peripheral Nervous System, which connects the Central Nervous System (the brain and spinal cord, housed within the skull and spine) with the tissues of the body, supplying those tissues with virtually all of their nerve control; and B, The Autonomic Nervous System, which controls the automatic, unconscious functions of the body, accounting primarily for the specific functions of the body's organs. The Autonomic system also includes 12 pairs of cranial nerves, which bypass the spinal cord, going directly from the brain to their target tissues, primarily structures of the head.

THE SPINAL COLUMN

The brain, spinal cord and spinal nerves are all extremely delicate structures. For this reason, Nature saw fit to protect this system as much as possible within the body's bony framework.

The brain is housed within the skull, a strong, bony protective armor. Similarly, the spinal column, or *spine*, is the home of the spinal cord, which is thereby afforded a protective bony housing. Figure 3 demonstrates this relationship.

In addition to protecting the spinal cord, the spine serves other important purposes. It is essentially the skeletal framework that keeps our bodies upright, like the steel frame of a building. Without it, our bodies would be amorphous, nonfunctional masses.

More than anything else, the spine is a dynamic structure. It is intimately involved in the dynamics of body movement, the result being that demands are perpetually made of it. Proper body mechanics depend heavily upon spinal flexibility and full, complete, harmonious movement of all the components of the spine. If ever spinal motion is impaired — and that happens far more commonly than you might think — the normal function of the body is disturbed in a variety of ways. Such malfunction can have serious far-reaching effects.

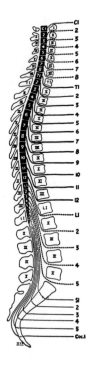

Figure 3. A lateral (side) view of the spine and spinal cord. The cord is housed within and protected by the bony spine, passing through the tunnel formed by the *posterior arches* of the vertebrae. It extends to the level of the second lumbar (low back) vertebra, giving rise to 31 pairs of spinal nerves, numbered sequentially according to the section of the spine (cervical, thoracic, lumbar, sacral) they emanate from.

The spine consists of twenty-four bones, called *vertebrae*. The vertebrae are separated from each other by cartilage cushions called *discs* (or "disks"), which are elastic, having about the same pliability as your ears or the tip of your nose. The discs provide flexibility and shock absorption for the spine. They also maintain the spaces between the vertebrae, which is necessary for undisturbed passage of the spinal nerves between the bones. Figure 4 demonstrates the relationship between the vertebrae and the spinal discs.

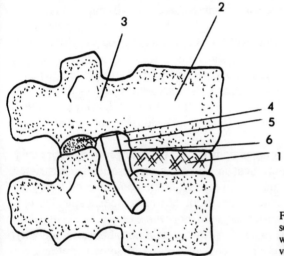

Figure 4. Two adjacent vertebrae separated by a disc (1). The weight-bearing front part of each vertebra is known as the *body* (2), with the rear section being known as the *posterior arch* (3). The vertebrae articulate on both the left and right sides of the arch (4) by the superior and inferior *articular processes*, as well as at the bodies, via the disc. The disc is a flexible shock-absorbing cushion that also serves the purpose of maintaining the space (the *foramen*) (5), for the *spinal nerve* (6) to pass through.

Ligaments, which can be likened to rubber bands, attach the spinal bones together, and cover a major portion of each surface — front, rear, sides — of each vertebra. The spinal ligaments are strong enough to maintain the integrity of the spine, and, normally, flexible enough to allow the full range of vertebral movement.

While there is some variation in the appearance of the bones of the spine, a typical vertebra possesses two basic parts: the front portion, or *body*, and the rear segment, called the *posterior arch*. The vertebral body is the weight-bearing portion of the bone, and the vertebral arches form a continuous tunnel that houses the spinal cord as it descends from the base of the brain.

The top and bottom surfaces of each vertebral body connect to the spinal disc above and below, while there are four small articulating surfaces (2 above, 2 below) on the posterior arch that connect each vertebra directly with the ones immediately above and below. There are, then, six joints associated with each vertebra. The plot thickens in the upper portion of the back, where each vertebra possesses two additional joints (one on each side) to receive a *rib*.

In order for the mechanics of body motion to occur properly, there must be full, free, harmonious movement in every one of these joints. Restricted mobility of any of the numerous spinal joints must be compensated for by the other joints and their supportive tissues. In other words, when a spinal joint is not fully mobile, adjacent segments begin to move *more than* or *differently from* the way they normally move, in an effort to maintain normal overall mobility. This compensatory reaction is a frequent cause of troublesome symptoms, not only of the back and neck, but of remote areas of the body as well.

It is the *muscles* of the back and neck that actually provide the movement of the spine. The various spinal muscles attach to specific locations on each vertebra, and the contraction of the muscles in various combinations accounts for the direction of spinal movement.

THE SPINAL DISCS

Each spinal disc has two components: an outer shell made of cartilage (a tough, elastic tissue) and an inner nucleus with the consistency of a gel. It is helpful to envision this structure as being similar in nature to a jelly doughnut. In its normal state, a disc is strong, pliable, and plush, and provides shock absorption, flexibility and spacing. Proper disc integrity is vital to normal spinal function.

Unlike most other tissues of the body, the discs receive no direct blood supply. This is significant because it is the blood that carries much-needed oxygen and nutrients to the tissues. To obtain these substances, the discs must rely on their inherent ability to imbibe body fluids that bathe them. This *imbibition* is made possible by a squeezing action that occurs during joint movement, in much the same way as squeezing a sponge allows fluid movement to occur. As long as the movement in a spinal joint is full and free, imbibition will maintain the normal integrity of the disc. If, however, mobility becomes impaired for any reason, disc integrity is compromised. If the situation persists for any length of time, the disc can become like a dried-up sponge: thin, brittle, and easily torn. You can imagine what would happen if you tried to bend a dry, brittle sponge. Obviously, it would tear, and the same thing can and does happen to spinal discs in that condition when a person happens to bend or twist in a way that stresses the disc beyond its ability to bend.

Such a situation, commonly referred to as a "slipped" disc, is more accurately termed a *ruptured* or torn disc. Whenever a ruptured disc is diagnosed — or whenever, in fact, a doctor points out a "degenerated" or "crushed" disc — the fact is that it has developed slowly as a product of this sequence of events. This is a perspective that is generally not taken by medical doctors, who seem to take the position that ruptured discs just suddenly "attack" people, in much the same way as other health problems just attack us.

Healthy spinal discs don't just degenerate or tear on their own, just as a healthy heart doesn't just suddenly stop working. You can be sure, when a disc problem develops, that the stage has been carefully set for it to occur.

SPINAL FIXATION

Restriction of spinal mobility is known as *fixation*. It is extremely common. In fact, most of us are walking around right now with fixations somewhere in our spines. You are not reading science fiction at this moment; you almost certainly have fixations in your spine as you read this. Figure 5 demonstrates a spinal fixation.

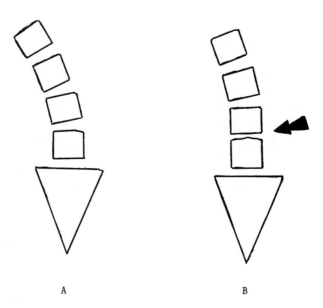

A   B

Figure 5. A, a diagram of normal spinal mobility, in which each joint is freely movable to the limits of its normal range of motion. B demonstrates a spinal fixation (arrow), in which the joint lacks proper mobility. Over time, the adjacent joints begin to compensate for the lost movement, and the immobile joint begins to demonstrate disc thinning and stiffening.

Often, fixation occurs with no outward symptoms. Nevertheless, its presence always compromises body function, and will eventually become symptomatic.

Primarily, it's a matter of mechanics. When your spine isn't working efficiently — i.e. when one or more of your spinal joints are not moving properly— the mechanics of your entire body become disturbed. In a very real sense, it is tantamount to having a machine with movable parts that aren't all moving. The works get "gummed-up," and proper function cannot possibly occur. Eventually, something has to give, and symptoms develop.

When one or more spinal joints are fixated (or more simply, "fixed"), adjacent ones compensate by working in a manner other than normal, which subjects their supportive muscles and ligaments to severe strain. As time goes by, symptoms of sprained or strained joints develop. These symptoms include local *pain, tenderness,* and eventually, more *restricted motion* (more fixation). Since spinal ligaments ultimately stiffen as a result of having been strained, the usual sequel to the compensatory strain is that the compensating joint eventually becomes fixed in position, which in turn causes compensation somewhere else, which produces still more fixation, and so on. The end result is an extremely stiff and immobile spine that develops with time. If that sounds familiar, it's not surprising. It's the picture of progressive stiffening that we generally consider to be an inevitable part of the aging process. The fact is, though, that it is not inevitable at all. Through chiropractic care, it's largely *preventable.*

THE VERTEBRAL SUBLUXATION COMPLEX

The clinical entity most commonly identified with the Chiropractic profession is a phenomenon known as the Vertebral Subluxation Complex, or simply, the *subluxation.*

A subluxation is defined as a displacement of a bone — usually a spinal bone — from its normal neutral position. A subluxation is something less than a "luxation" (dislocation), in which the bone is displaced outside its normal range of motion. In other words, a subluxated vertebra is misaligned, but still within its range of motion.

A spinal joint must be evaluated in terms of its dynamic function rather than its static position. A subluxation will primarily occur if (a) the muscles pulling on the bone are unbalanced, causing it to deviate from its normal position,

(b) one or more of the spinal ligaments lack proper flexibility, causing the joint to be fixated in an abnormal position, at least during certain movements, or (c) the joint's ligaments have become excessively flexible due to injury or compensation for nearby fixations, in turn causing the bone to deviate from its normal relative position. In any case, the problem is a dynamic one, since muscles and ligaments are functional components of the joint.

Subluxations, then, can involve joints that are either *hypomobile* (fixated) or *hypermobile* (compensating). A fixated spinal joint may be immobile in all directions of potential movement, or only in one direction, depending upon which and how many ligaments have lost their elasticity. The bone may be "stuck" in its normal neutral position, or it may be misaligned (subluxated). A hypermobile subluxation involves joint instability and vacillation of position.

Although Organized Medicine disparages the importance of the vertebral subluxation, it is not a figment of a fertile chiropractic imagination. It is a significant clinical entity, with very definite biomechanical consequences, and — perhaps even more importantly — remote organic effects as well.

The Vertebral Subluxation Complex has several components, including those that are biomechanical, physiological, neurological, and pathological. Even when there are no noticeable symptoms, these factors are involved in setting the stage for problems to occur.

The major *biomechanical* aspects of subluxation have already been mentioned, including both fixation and hypermobility. Biomechanical impairment leads to tissue changes and eventual symptoms.

Some of the changes are *physiological* in nature. Ligament tissue becomes less elastic. Ligaments and muscles in *adjacent* joints become strained, resulting in *inflammation*, which produces *pain*.

Various *neurological* changes occur. Transmission of the pain signals resulting from inflammation is one example of altered nerve impulses. These signals result in a subsequent barrage of nerve signals that produce *muscle spasm* (another physiological change), which further impairs movement (biomechanical). Additional neurological changes may be the result of a nerve becoming either *pinched* or *inflamed* as it exits between the vertebrae, the product of either the aberrant motion or the inflammatory process occurring in the joint. Nerve involvement can also take the form of *pressure from a bulging disc*, the result of joint imbalance. Figure 6 demonstrates how a spinal nerve can be pinched by either a disc or vertebra.

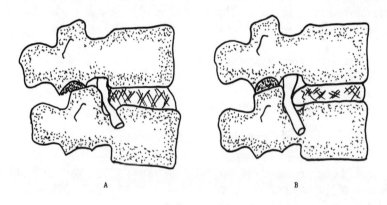

Figure 6. A, a vertebral misalignment (subluxation) causing nerve compression, and B, a bulging disc compressing a spinal nerve.

Nerve root compression or inflammation can cause severe symptoms, both locally and remotely. *Local symptoms* may include pain, tenderness, numbness, and tingling. *Remote symptoms* may be either *musculoskeletal* (involving the trunk and extremities) or *organic*.

Musculoskeletal symptoms can include pain, numbness, tingling, or weakness (even to the point of paralysis, as in the case of Frank, the shop teacher), and typically occur in the arms and legs. *Organic symptoms* can also occur, because of the relationship between spinal nerves and organ function. Chest or abdominal pain, indigestion, and symptoms of asthma may all be the result of spinal subluxation.

Or, there may be no symptoms at all, while organic disease develops silently. One or more organs may begin to function somewhat sluggishly — say, only 80% of normal — but continue to perform well enough for you to "get by" without symptoms. The body is such a remarkable compensating machine that you may go for months or even years with no symptoms of malfunction, all the while thinking that you are "healthy." Sooner or later, though — when the organ is severely enough impaired — your body will start sending signals.

That is the *pathological* component of the Vertebral Subluxation Complex. When an organ's nerve supply is compromised over a long enough period of time, disease will develop. Once the organ begins to malfunction, the disease process will proceed exactly like a disease caused in any other way.

THE WINDSOR REPORT

Although research is currently underway to provide indisputable evidence of the link between spinal subluxation and organic pathology, such evidence was actually reported a long time ago.

As long ago as 1921, Dr. Henry Windsor, a medical doctor at the University of Pennsylvania, took a special interest in the relationship between spinal nerve interference and organic disease. In one study, Dr. Windsor reported his findings after dissecting 50 human cadavers.

Among the 50 bodies, he discovered 139 organs that had been diseased at the time of death. Quite obviously, the organic disease could be said to have contributed to death in most of the cases.

Dr. Windsor then proceeded to trace the nerve supply to each organ from the point at which it entered the organ all the way back to its exit from the spine. His findings were revealing: in *138* of the cases, Dr. Windsor found spinal derangements (subluxations) at the level of the spine giving rise to the nerves to the diseased organs.

Based on his findings, his logical conclusion was that *spinal derangements affect spinal nerve function and can contribute to the development of organic disease, which ultimately causes death.*

Taking Dr. Windsor's conclusions one step futher, one could say that *correcting* and/or *preventing* spinal subluxations can restore proper nerve function, thereby preventing organic disease and prolonging life. While difficult to prove, it is a very plausible theory that cannot be disproven. Since chiropractors devote most of their time and energy to the very endeavor of correcting subluxations and fixations, it may turn out in the final analysis that Chiropractic's greatest contribution to mankind is to prevent disease and prolong life in this manner.

DR. CHUNG SUH

One of the biggest single sources of contemporary research into the effect of spinal subluxations is Chung H. Suh, PhD, at the University of Colorado. A specialist in spinal biomechanics, Dr. Suh has demonstrated conclusively that "the vertebral subluxation is very real. We have documented it again and again. With this scientific documentation, no one can dispute the existence of vertebral subluxation." He has further stated that "Vertebral Subluxation Complex changes the entire health of the body. This has been proven many times. The spine is not an isolated structure.... We have proved that V.S.C. causes not only structural dysfunction of the spine and adjacent tissues, but it also causes nerve dysfunction."

Thanks in large part to the efforts of Dr. Suh, it continues to become clearer and clearer that vertebral subluxations and fixations play a significant role in the causation of troublesome health problems, both biomechanical and organic in nature.

OTHER RELATED RESEARCH

There is currently a great deal more research being conducted into the nature and significance of spinal subluxations and fixations, as well as the short- and long-term effects of chiropractic spinal treatments. One of the problems that has stood in the way of large-scale chiropractic research has been a lack of government funding for such projects (yet another consequence of the AMA's stance on Chiropractic and the general bias it has generated). While some funding has now become available, the lion's share of money for chiropractic research continues to come from private donations. As a result, the scope and magnitude of such projects has necessarily been limited.

There is research being conducted at several of the chiropractic colleges in this country that can be expected to yield revealing results as time goes by. In addition, there are numerous sub-specialty groups and institutes that have been established in the Chiropractic field for the purpose of conducting research in particular aspects of chiropractic therapy. Included among these are the International College of Applied Kinesiology, the Motion Palpation Institute, Activator Methods, Inc., the Sacro-Occipital Research Society International, and more. There is also an organization called The Foundation for Chiropractic Education and Research that is involved with ongoing research in Chiropractic.

It won't be long before these research efforts are able to demonstrate conclusively what practicing chiropractors know from experience: that spinal fixations and subluxations are significant clinical entities, and that chiropractic treatment is extremely effective for the correction of such problems, thereby relieving their related conditions, and very possibly preventing disease and prolonging life.

WHY DO FIXATIONS AND SUBLUXATIONS DEVELOP?

After learning about the nature of fixations and subluxations, patients frequently ask the question, "*How in the world* did I get something like *that*?" Once you understand how and why these entities develop, the far more logical question is, "How in the world can anyone *avoid* them?"

Fixations and subluxations of the spine are the natural result of all the wear and tear, stress, abuse, and demands to which the spine is exposed over a lifetime. Such stress is cumulative, the product of an ongoing process that begins earlier in life than you might think.

The very first source of spinal stress is the birth process itself. When a baby begins to descend from the womb, what is the first thing the doctor does? He or she grasps the baby's head and *twists* the child by the neck in order to accommodate the shoulders in the birth canal. At the same time, the doctor *pulls* the baby outward and into the world. The amount of force utilized in this combined twisting and pulling procedure is often quite severe. That amount of force applied to the well-developed spinal tissues of an adult is often sufficient to injure those tissues. Just imagine the effect it can have on a newborn, whose spinal ligaments and muscles are not yet equal to the task of supporting and affording protection for the structure of the spine.

That, as it turns out, is only the beginning. The insults and abuse suffered by the spine continue to mount as time goes by. A parent who, while holding a baby, turns suddenly in response to a voice or another signal, can traumatize a child's spine. The baby's body goes along with the parent's turning motion, but the head is left behind, pulling up the rear. The result is not unlike a "whiplash" injury suffered by a passenger in an automobile that is suddenly hit from behind.

There's more yet. As the child begins to ambulate, he or she suffers all kinds of spinal insults. A fall from a sofa, a crawling collision with a coffee table, a tumble down a flight of stairs; you name it, and it is probably a source of spinal stress. Infants and toddlers are resilient, thank goodness; but the little spinal insults leave their mark.

As a child grows, and his or her activities become a little more rough-and-tumble, the assault on the spine continues. We have all had the experience of sitting on a see-saw, when suddenly and without warning, the boy or girl on the other end has made the decision to abandon ship. That jolt to the spine, forgotten moments later, leaves an enduring signature. Childhood games, while chock full of redeeming qualities, all produce spinal insult.

When this author was a boy growing up on the streets of New York City, one of the most popular games was known as "Johnny-Ride-A-Pony." The game was played by two teams, usually consisting of about four or five players apiece. One team, the "pony," would form a human horse: the head player would stand, back to a building wall, cradling the head and shoulders of the next player, who was bent from the waist, waiting to receive someone on his back; each successive player then bent over in turn, arms and hands wrapped around the waist and hips of the previous player. The finished product of this endeavor was a long "horse" awaiting its rider, "Johnny." The team that was Johnny would line up several yards to the rear of the pony. One at a time, the players would run and pounce on the horse, with the ultimate objective of causing its collapse. If they succeeded, they were the winners of that round. If the horse survived the assault, that team was the victor.

If ever a game was invented that was a chiropractor's (and a spine-owner's) nightmare, that was it. Here again, though, none of us ever felt ill effects back then; the price is paid years later, in the form of chronic fixations and subluxations that rear their ugly heads.

Adulthood offers little relief. Most people become more sedentary as adults, providing the spinal tissues with insufficient exercise to keep them strong and supple. Spinal ligaments and muscles, responding to "the law of supply and demand," become increasingly weak, stiff, and rigid from the lack of vigorous activity. At the same time, however, they are being asked to do the job of supporting our day-to-day activities, such as bending, twisting, lifting, and the like. Even the sedentary spine is under great stress, and — with spinal ligaments and muscles not kept strong and pliable — begins to demonstrate the telltale aches and pains. Frequently, the "straw that breaks the camel's back" (the reader will please excuse the pun) is the occasional vigorous activity or chore, such as moving furniture or lifting a heavy object. Back muscles and ligaments may tear, and even the disc may become torn, if the stage has been methodically set for it to happen.

Getting back to the original question, *that* is "how in the world" fixations and subluxations develop, and why the real question is how they can be avoided.

Spinal fixations and subluxations, forever ignored by the medical community, constitute the realm in which the Chiropractic profession makes its singular contribution to health and well being. Given the overwhelming clinical evidence and the ever-increasing research evidence of the existence and significance of these clinical entities, it is astonishing that such a gap exists in the way in which they are regarded by the Medical and Chiropractic professions. The fact that such a gap exists is further testimony to medical shortsightedness.

6 Chiropractic Practice

The doctor of the future will give no medicine, but will interest his patients in the care of the human frame, in diet, and in the cause and prevention of disease.

Thomas A. Edison

Chiropractors were the original "wholistic" physicians. Long before the term became popular, chiropractors were concerning themselves with preventive health care and all of the factors that influenced a patient's health. Another way of saying it is that chiropractors look for the reasons a person's symptoms developed — the particular combination of systemic stress and malfunction, together with environmental and lifestyle factors — and work to eliminate those problems, while most medical physicians want to give a patient something to take for the headache, something for the sniffles, something for the stomach upset, and so on. In yet other words, the chiropractor treats the person and not the disease.

This approach to health care is of tremendous importance. The chiropractor's role is a critical one, in that few other practitioners address the whole person, and no others address the vitally important issue of spinal function. In a world of cover-up drugs and needless and useless surgery, there is a great need for a broader general understanding and appreciation of this remarkable specialty.

THE CHIROPRACTIC ADJUSTMENT

By far, the single most unique, important and common element of chiropractic health care is that procedure known as the *chiropractic adjustment*. The adjustment is a technique of physical manipulation of the spine applied with the objective of mobilizing a fixated joint. The adjustment is a gentle, yet dynamic thrust applied to a particular spinal joint in such a way as to generate movement in a specific direction. Basically, it is an attempt to "coax" a restricted joint to begin moving. Applied repeatedly over a period of time, spinal adjustments are capable of restoring mobility to even the most chronic spinal fixations. Deep-rooted fixations that have existed for several years typically require months of care. Fixations of lesser duration and severity respond in less time. A recent, mild fixation will often respond in as little as one treatment.

It is important to remember that spinal fixation is an ongoing *process* that must be arrested, reversed, and corrected. Treatment, then, must also be a process. The chiropractor's recommendation for treatment is based upon the specific nature and history of the condition in each case. Chronic, long-term fixations and subluxations may need to be adjusted several times a week for a number of weeks, followed by gradually diminishing frequency of care, to properly and effectively encourage the changes that are desired. Acute, painful conditions need to be handled in stages. Most often, the pain and inflammation of tissue injury must first be treated with ice and physiotherapy for a period of time before attempts can be made to correct the spinal malfunction responsible for the condition. Such acute case management is typically carried out on a daily basis at first, until the symptoms subside and adjustments can be administered several times a week. Milder conditions, of course, require a lesser frequency and a shorter duration of care.

Since many patients only seek chiropractic care after progressive degeneration of spinal joints has already begun, some conditions cannot be totally corrected. Even in such cases, however, there is reason to be optimistic. Despite the fact that medical literature essentially states that degenerative conditions are irreversible, that is not necessarily so. I have seen cases in which post-treatment X-rays have demonstrated a return to normal thickness and flexibility in discs that had previously been "degenerated." Restoring joint mobility through chiropractic spinal adjustments has, in these cases, effectively restored the ability of the spinal discs to imbibe body fluids and become fully functional. In any case, even when full disc integrity cannot be restored, chiropractic treatment can usually improve function and relieve discomfort.

Chiropractors primarily evaluate and restore spinal biomechanics. While symptoms are, naturally, important to a chiropractor, he or she pays far greater attention to spinal dynamics and the application of treatment to restore normal mobility. The chiropractor considers his or her job done when spinal motion is fully restored, and not just when symptoms have abated. Usually, symptoms respond well before total correction has occurred, and more treatment is necessary for full functional restoration. The objective should always be total correction.

Because of our society's "crisis medicine" orientation, it is not uncommon for a patient to want to stop care when symptoms disappear. That is, of course, the patient's prerogative, but it is important to understand that until the spinal malfunction is fully corrected, there is still a substantial vulnerability for the condition to recur. More accurately, *the condition never really goes away* — only the symptoms do. But as long as the spinal malfunction continues to exist to some extent, it undermines body function and health, and will ultimately cause symptoms once again. The best way to prevent recurrence is to continue with chiropractic care until the doctor is satisfied that correction has been made.

Chiropractic works on two levels. First, chiropractic adjustments restore proper mechanics of the spine, which enhances joint function, corrects specific joint problems, and prevents injury due to improper spinal dynamics. It is this facet of chiropractic care that principally affects problems that are *muscloskeletal* in nature.

Secondly, because of the relationship between spinal nerves and organ function, the removal of nerve interference by the correction of spinal fixations and subluxations enhances organ function and health in general. To the extent that it does that, I believe that Chiropractic can prevent disease and prolong life.

For these reasons, everybody walking the face of this planet should have regular, periodic chiropractic care to improve and maintain proper spinal function.

CHIROPRACTIC MAINTENANCE CARE

Because the stresses and demands that produce spinal impairment are constant and ongoing, chiropractors recommend that patients return periodically for evaluation and treatment of spinal and body mechanics. Such *maintenance* visits are not unlike taking your car to be "tuned up" periodically. Maintenance care constitutes an ongoing program of preventive care, primarily addressing the structural component of disease causation, and ensuring against troublesome and debilitating spinal-related problems.

People who follow these recommendations are taking responsibility for their own well-being, rather than leaving it up to Fate, Chance, or their doctor. They are acknowledging that health problems don't just "attack," but are the result of an ongoing process. Such individuals tend to experience a lower incidence of recurrence of their problems, as well as a generally enhanced level of well-being.

Many chiropractic patients realize that such a problem of chiropractic maintenance care would be equally valuable for friends and relatives, even though they may not suffer from symptoms that might prompt them to seek care, and refer these people for treatment. Such a referred patient is fortunate indeed; he or she probably doesn't even realize the favor that has been done by the caring friend or family member who made the suggestion.

EXERCISE ALONE WON'T DO IT

Some people have the mistaken notion that flexibility exercises can take the place of chiropractic spinal adjustments. While it seems like a reasonable idea, the fact is that exercise alone is not capable of eliminating joint fixations and subluxations.

Stretching exercises work *entire sections* of the spine rather than individual spinal joints. There is no exercise that can work just a single spinal joint, since the muscles involved are large ones that each attach to several vertebrae.

Because of this, those joints that are mobile will move during a specific exercise, and those that are fixated will not. The result will be an *aggravation* of the problem, since it is the *compensating joints* that will be doing the work, and not those that need mobilizing.

Once, however, the spine has been properly mobilized by chiropractic adjustments, exercise is absolutely essential for maintenance of proper function. The chiropractor will recommend specific exercises during the latter stages of care to enhance and hasten full recovery. In addition, the doctor will more than likely suggest an exercise program along with a program of maintenance treatments. By so doing, the doctor and patient are maximizing the opportunity for optimal spinal function and minimizing the likelihood that problems will develop.

EXTRA-SPINAL ADJUSTMENTS

The spine is only one part of the biomechanical structure of the human body. There are numerous other movable joints, each one subjected to demands similar to those placed on the spine, and each one capable of malfunctioning. The chiropractor considers and evaluates each of these movable parts in the evaluation of a patient's condition and overall body dynamics, and frequently performs adjustments in these areas as well as in the spine.

Most notable among these joints are the *sacroiliac joints* of the pelvis. Situated just below the spine — and demarcated by two dimples just below and to either side of the lowest spinal joint — the sacroiliacs are intimately involved in spinal dynamics. Functionally, in fact, they can be considered to be a part of the spine.

The sacroiliac joints function under a great deal of stress, largely for two reasons. First of all, they bear the weight of the entire upper half of the body, and they do so at a precarious angle that subjects them to intense gravitational pressure. Secondly, demands are made of them in just about every movement of the body, so they are almost constantly required to be in action (Figure 7).

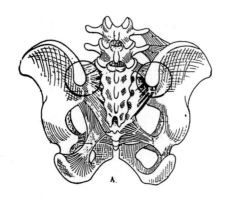

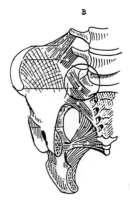

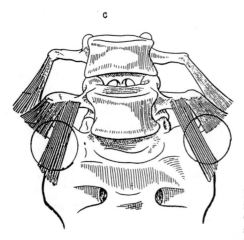

Figure 7. A, rear view of sacroiliac joints (circled), and B and
C, front views of sacroiliacs,
showing some of the many
supportive ligaments.

As a result of all these demands, the ligaments of the sacroiliacs — just like those in the spine — frequently become strained. If injured sufficiently, they can be the cause of varying degrees of low back pain, and can also be involved in *sciatica* (pain in the leg). If the strain is more subtle, it may not be symptomatic, but the healing ligaments may become increasingly stiff and rigid. Fixations of the sacroiliac joints are perhaps the most common in the body, and can be at the root of a variety of painful conditions by virtue of the compensation they produce in the spine. Perhaps as many as 75% of chiropractic patients, regardless of where they hurt, have some degree of fixation of the sacroiliac joints that may be directly related to their symptoms.

Other joints play a role in body mechanics and must, therefore, be considered as well by the chiropractor. Specifically, the *hips, knees, ankles, shoulders, elbows,* and *wrists* may be mechanically impaired and in need of treatment. Chiropractic manipulation of these joints may correct painful conditions involving them or conditions elsewhere in which they play a role.

The feet also play an important role in the support and ambulation of the body, since they are the platform upon which we stand and walk. The feet and ankles are frequently adjusted by the chiropractor. In addition, a patient may be in need of postural foot supports known as *orthotics*, which restore balance to feet chronically subjected to the effects of wear and tear. Many chiropractors will refer a patient with such a need to a *podiatrist* for this service, although some prefer to provide the service themselves.

PHYSICAL THERAPY

The majority of chiropractors utilize various types of physiotherapy equipment in patient care. Some types of therapy are very effective in the reduction of pain and inflammation in acute conditions, while others are more valuable for restoring tissue integrity and function in chronic conditions. If a patient's needs for therapy cannot be met in the chiropractor's office, the person will be referred to a physical therapist for the most effective care. Physical therapy generally expedites both symptomatic relief and the ultimate correction of a patient's condition.

SPINAL DISC CONDITIONS

Chiropractic treatment is often extremely effective for conditions involving spinal discs. Even those cases in which discs have already been diagnosed as "slipped," "ruptured," "torn," or "prolapsed," and in need of surgery may often respond to care.

Only about 10 to 15% of all conditions that demonstrate the classic symptoms of disc involvement — intense back or neck pain; pain, numbness or tingling in an arm, buttock or leg; and *antalgia* (a distortion of body position in which the body instinctively leans away from pain) — actually involve discs that are damaged in such a way that surgery may be required. Despite the sophistication of today's diagnostic procedures, none of them are infallible in the determination and estimation of disc damage. Although "CAT" scans are quite effective, neither they nor myelograms are foolproof, and so evidence of disc damage may be suggestive at best. In many of these cases, surgery is recommended by the medical physician solely on the basis of presumptive evidence and in the absence of any viable medical options.

In such cases, surgery is often performed unnecessarily. Conservative chiropractic care may very well have been able to correct the condition in many such cases, thereby obviating the need for surgery. A surgical procedure is only the answer in the small percentage of cases in which the disc is damaged beyond the body's ability to repair it. For all other cases, Chiropractic should be tried before the person submits to surgery.

Chiropractors routinely treat patients for whom surgery has already been recommended, and some for whom it has actually already been scheduled. A great many of these patients recover completely and never need the surgery. Of course, it doesn't always happen that way. Sometimes, a disc is actually ruptured beyond repair, in which case chiropractic adjustments are not going to be effective. But, in all but the most obvious and painful cases, there is nothing to be lost by trying a program of conservative care. It will do no harm, and — unlike surgery — nothing about it is irreversible. An experienced and conscientious chiropractor will recognize when a condition isn't responding as it should, and will refer the patient for more appropriate care.

OTHER TYPICAL CHIROPRACTIC CONDITIONS

Since the majority of body functions are controlled or monitored wholly or partly via the spinal cord, there is almost no limit to the types of conditions that may respond to chiropractic care. Certain conditions, however, lend themselves better than others to chiropractic correction, and typify the majority of problems seen daily in chiropractic offices. Such conditions include: *headache*; *pain in the neck*; *pain, numbness or tingling in one or both legs (sciatica); arthritis; bursitis; tendinitis and back pain.*

Certain organic conditions often respond readily to chiropractic treatment. One possible cause of the symptoms of *asthma* is interference with the nerve supply to the lungs. In those cases, symptoms typically abate totally in response to a short program of spinal adjustments. Bear in mind, however, that not all cases of asthma have their roots at the spine. But those cases that do emanate from the spine respond readily and often miraculously to chiropractic adjustments. Other organic conditions known to respond to care include structurally-induced heart and chest pain, digestive upset (if the nerve supply to the stomach or intestines is compromised, digestive glands may secrete in altered quantities, and the resultant tissue irritation may result in an *ulcer*), and menstrual cramps. Practically any symptom of practically any body part could be the result of spinal subluxation, and may very well respond to chiropractic care.

So-called "whiplash" injuries should be almost the exclusive domain of the chiropractic physician. Whiplash involves severe strain and tearing of supportive spinal muscles and ligaments. When they heal, there is bound to be significant spinal fixation unless proper care is applied, preferably from the beginning. Injured ligaments lose flexibility and must be treated methodically to gradually restore lost mobility.

The usual medical approach to such problems is to utilize a cervical collar, pain-killing medication, rest and physical therapy. This regimen will allow nature to heal the injured tissue, but overlooks the most important element — joint mobilization — and will ensure residual fixation and lifelong problems of a chronic, progressive nature. Chiropractic care, on the other hand, will allow normal mobility to be gradually restored as the tissues heal, with virtually no residual involvement in the majority of cases. Instead of a lifetime of chronic, progressive neck problems, a whiplash victim who receives chiropractic treatments can look forward to a total recovery in most cases.

TYPES OF CHIROPRACTIC PROCEDURES

There are numerous and varied chiropractic treatment techniques, and each chiropractor has his or her favorites. They all work, and you should trust your chiropractor's judgment in the selection of procedures used in your therapy.

The chiropractic adjustment is usually performed by hand. However, the use of mechanical adjusting instruments is growing. The most common of these, known as an *Activator*, is a hand-held device that is spring-loaded and resembles a dental impactor. The use of mechanical adjusting devices such as the Activator ensures consistency and effectively alleviates apprehension in patients who are uncomfortable with the manual procedures.

Another common method of treatment involves a discipline known as *Applied Kinesiology (A.K.)*. "Kinesiology" is the study of body movement and muscle function. *Applied* Kinesiology is a system of diagnosis and treatment that utilizes relationships between muscles and body balance and between muscles and organs, and involves the testing of muscles for their relative strength.

The utilization of this procedure enables the doctor to gain important information about body balance and function that would be otherwise inaccessible. While still in its early stages as far as widespread utilization goes, A.K. will one day prove to be of tremendous clinical importance.

The chiropractic technique of evaluating the dynamics of joint function is known as *motion palpation*, and involves pressure-testing the spinal joints for their level of pliability. A well-trained motion palpator can easily feel the degree of mobility in a joint and determine where fixation exists. The Motion

Palpation Institute of Huntington Beach, California has compiled a vast library of research studies relating to spinal and pelvic joint mobility, and has developed a very effective teaching format as a result.

Another extremely effective chiropractic technique is known as *Sacro-Occipital Therapy*, and involves relationships among the bones of the skull and pelvis. S.O.T techniques have demonstrated how distortion and fixation of those bones can cause a variety of conditions by affecting the flow of *cerebrospinal fluid*, and have achieved remarkable results in treatment. S.O.T., like the other techniques that have been highlighted, is truly a specialty within the Chiropractic profession and takes years to learn fully.

There are numerous other specific chiropractic techniques and areas of specialization, and each is effective in its own way. Most chiropractors have a general knowledge of several of the different techniques, while many limit their work to the use of just one. Here again, if you get a good feeling about your doctor, trust his or her judgement, and the results will most likely justify your confidence.

WHOLISTIC CARE

As mentioned earlier, chiropractors were the original *wholistic* (holistic) physicians. Wholistic health care is an approach to the care of a patient that considers all factors of the person's health and lifestyle, and involves treatment of the "whole person" as he or she relates to his or her environment. More simply stated, wholistic care involves treating the person rather than the symptoms, and typically involves addressing factors such as diet, nutritional supplementation, exercise, stress management, and habit patterns.

Most chiropractors utilize the wholistic approach to patient care. In discussing a person's health history, the doctor will want to learn as much as possible about each of those factors that affect the person's health. Armed with this knowledge, the chiropractor customarily makes recommendations involving these factors that will not only influence the person's response to treatment for the painful condition at hand, but can have a profound effect on the patient's general health and well-being as well.

Certainly, the chiropractor has an interest in relieving the symptoms that brought the patient in the door, but that is only the tip of the iceberg. To the extent that the patient is also interested, the chiropractor's prime concern is that person's overall health. Once that is understood, the patient's ultimate objective often changes, and patient and doctor become aligned in looking at the "big picture." This scenario is the epitome of health care.

THE CHIROPRACTIC EXAMINATION

Like any other physician, the chiropractor utilizes the gamut of diagnostic procedures available for the evaluation of a patient's physical health. Whatever procedures are necessary to properly determine the nature of a particular problem will be employed. Typical chiropractic examination procedures include: a standard *physical examination*, including evaluation of vital signs such as blood pressure, pulse rate, and the like; *orthopedic and neurological testing*, to determine the nature and extent of joint, muscle and nerve involvement; *laboratory tests* (i.e., blood tests), whenever necessary, to evaluate systemic health; *X-rays* in most cases, to give the doctor a bird's-eye view of the spine and its supportive structures; and, when absolutely necessary, referral for such studies as CAT scans and Magnetic Resonance Imaging. In each case, the doctor wants to compile all the information necessary to properly evaluate the situation.

Where the chiropractic approach differs markedly from that of the medical doctor is in relation to the emphasis placed on *biomechanics*. Whereas the MD wishes merely to rule out fracture, dislocation, or pathology, the chiropractor doesn't end there. In fact, that's just the beginning. The chiropractic examination includes an evaluation of the spine and pelvis in *static and dynamic function*. The chiropractor will most often push, pull, and turn the patient in various directions while simultaneously feeling the response of individual spinal and pelvic joints. This technique, referred to earlier as *motion palpation*, enables the doctor to gain an accurate sense of the relative mobility of each joint. Much of the recommended treatment program is predicated upon this evaluation.

CHIROPRACTIC PRACTICE

Chiropractic X-rays usually differ from medical X-rays in that (1) they are most often taken with the patient in the standing position, rather than lying down, so that the effects of posture and gravity can be properly taken into consideration (since they generally play a significant role in the cause of a person's problem); and (2) they are often done utilizing positions that demonstrate the absence or presence of joint motion. Pictures taken in different bending positions can be infinitely more valuable than neutral ones in that regard. When you think about it, it makes a world of sense: when a person is suffering from a mechanical problem of the spine, how could it possibly be detected with the patient at rest, lying supine on a table, the way all such medical X-rays are taken? The answer is, it can't. The effects of posture, gravity, and movement have all been eliminated from such a study, making it impossible for the doctor to properly evaluate the patient's condition. Of course, since spinal mechanics are the farthest thing from the medical doctor's mind, such a logical study of spinal dynamics is never considered.

The fact is, whenever a painful condition of the neck or back doesn't involve a fracture, dislocation, or pathological condition, it is virtually always a mechanical disturbance that is causing the problem. The chiropractor is the only health professional who has been properly trained to evaluate and treat these conditions. In contrast to the chiropractor's approach of restoring proper function, the usual medical alternative is bedrest, medication, and physical therapy. There is no comparison.

THE NEW ZEALAND REPORT

In 1978, a commission was formed in New Zealand specifically to determine whether Chiropractic care should be covered by the national health insurance. After a thorough and comprehensive investigation, the commission conclude, among other things, that:

> Chiropractors carry out spinal diagnosis and therapy
> on a sophisticated level . . . .

91

Chiropractors are the only health practitioners who are necessarily equipped by their education and training to carry out spinal manual therapy . . . .

General medical practitioners and physiotherapists have no adequate training in spinal manual therapy, though a few have acquired skill in it subsequent to graduation . . . .

The education and training of a registered chiropractor are sufficient to enable him to determine whether there are contra-indications to spinal manual therapy in a particular case, and whether the patient should have medical care instead of or as well as chiropractic care.

CHIROPRACTIC AND SPORTS

Chiropractic and sports together constitute a perfect match. Obviously, athletic activities involve body mechanics. An athlete relies upon proper dynamics of body movement for optimal performance. Chiropractic restores and maintains proper dynamics of motion. What could be a more suitable combination?

Chiropractic care can improve athletic performance by enhancing joint function. An athlete's body is like a finely-tuned machine: the more optimally its parts are moving together, the more efficient will be its performance. In athletic competition, where the difference between victory and defeat is measured in inches or split seconds, relative body mechanics can make the difference.

Regular chiropractic adjustments can further help the athlete by aiding in the prevention of injury. Strains, sprains, and other common athletic injuries are often caused by faulty joint mobility. A joint in which there is restricted movement will not only be more easily sprained, but it will place increased demands on other joints by forcing them to compensate, rendering them more susceptible to injury as well. A regular program of chiropractic treatments can reduce the likelihood of injury by keeping the joints mobile.

Improved performance and prevention of injuries — what better combination could one ask for in the athletic arena? Across the board, every athletic team, from junior high school up through college and professional sports, should have a team chiropractor. Some do, but that is far too often the result of toilsome campaigning on the part of an enthusiastic coach who has had the opportunity to personally witness Chiropractic's effectiveness. Far more commonly, negative bias on the part of team or school officials denies the athletes such benefits.

The United States Olympic team has, however, been including chiropractors on the medical staff since 1980. This can be directly attributed to the lobbying efforts of the athletes, who have long demanded Chiropractic's presence at competitions.

Numerous athletic careers have been saved and lengthened by chiropractic care. More often, however, promising careers are impaired or cut short by disabling back ailments for which chiropractic care is never sought. Every serious athlete, whether a sufferer of such problems or not, should seek the benefits of chiropractic treatment for the relief and/or prevention of such debilitating problems, as well as to maximize performance.

CORPORATE CHIROPRACTIC

The company for which you work is another team that should have an official team chiropractor. Chiropractic care can increase employee productivity in a variety of ways.

In the treatment of industrial back injuries, statistics clearly demonstrate that chiropractic treatment is typically able to get the employee back to work in less time, at lower cost, and with a lower incidence of recurrence than medical care for the same condition. Nationwide, billions of dollars could probably be saved from that point of view alone if every company had its own chiropractor.

On a broader basis, for the treatment of a wide variety of nagging, troublesome conditions that limit worker effectiveness, chiropractic care made available to employees on a routine basis can reduce work days lost to illness, injury and malaise. Nagging headaches, neck pain and stiffness, upper back pain and tension — problems that frequently cause employees to leave work early, stay out for several days, or at least be totally nonproductive on the job — often respond immediately and completely to just a single chiropractic adjustment.

In a California workmen's compensation study involving 1,000 cases, it was found that workers who received chiropractic care were able to return to work in an average of 15.6 days, as compared to an average of 32 days for workers with similar injuries who received only medical care. Other studies have produced similar findings, both in workman's compensation and non-work-related cases, and chiropractic patients observe day-in and day-out the beneficial effects of treatment for their nagging, tension-related conditions.

In terms of prevention, regular chiropractic treatments for the purpose of health maintenance could very possibly reduce the incidence of illness, enhance employee well-being, and thereby dramatically increase productivity. Fewer days will likely be lost to illness (both *saving* the company money AND *making* the company money), morale will be higher (a proven money-maker), and employees will be more alert, dynamic and productive. And, their increased level of alertness can help prevent on-the-job injuries caused by carelessness and fatigue.

THE DOCTOR OF THE FUTURE

It is interesting to note the uncanny accuracy of two quotations previously referred to in this book. The first, attributed to Hippocrates, the "Father of Medicine," advises the physician, "In all disease, look first to the spine." Hippocrates, without the benefit of thousands of years of documented medical history and research or the sophisticated procedures available to today's physician, was still able to discern and axiomize this truth.

And Thomas A. Edison, hardly a medical man but certainly a man of logic and science — and one with more than a passing interest in the nature of electrical impulses — predicted that the "doctor of the future" will be one who pays attention to "the care of the human frame," as well as "in diet and in the cause and prevention of disease." It is also useful to note that he characterized such a physician as being one who "gives no medicine" as well.

More and more, we hear voices within the medical profession echoing and concurring with the chiropractic claim that spinal subluxations and fixations are not only a frequent cause of back- and neck-related problems, but the cause of many organic conditions as well. As of this writing, such sentiments are more commonly heard in Europe, where there seems to be a good deal more emphasis on manual medicine and attention paid to the spine.

As time goes by, the health care community and the general public will come to realize the sagacity of the points of view proffered by such scientists as Hippocrates and Edison. At the same time, both groups will come to recognize not only the validity, but the *preeminence* of the Chiropractic approach to health care.

7

So, Where's the Beef?

SO, WHERE'S THE BEEF?

At this point, it would be reasonable for you to be wondering why anyone would be opposed to Chiropractic. After all, it's certainly a logical, rational and sensible approach to health care.

You can rest assured, however, that there is plenty of opposition to Chiropractic. Every chiropractor encounters it in some form every day. Whether it's in an attitude or sentiment expressed by a patient, another professional, or an insurance representative, nary a day goes by in the life of a chiropractor when he or she doesn't hear at least one example of bias against the profession. The source of the bias, as it turns out, is also the source of the widespread fear, apprehension, and misunderstanding about Chiropractic.

Opposition to Chiropractic comes primarily from a single source — the medical profession. Now, that statement needs clarification. The actual source of the antipathy is not the individual medical doctor, although he or she is most often caught up in it.

That is to say, medical doctors are commonly antagonistic toward Chiropractic; but when they are, it is rarely on the basis of any personal knowledge or experience regarding the profession.

Most medical doctors have little knowledge about Chiropractic. Whatever feelings they may have about it have been derived from what they have been taught or what they have read in medical publications on the subject. Unfortunately for them, for the Chiropractic profession, and for the public, the information they receive is generally slanted, biased, misleading and inaccurate. As a result, the average MD has a decidedly negative opinion of Chiropractic, but one that isn't based on the facts.

In fairness to these doctors, they really can't be faulted for their opinion, because they're merely reacting to what they've been led to believe as fact. They are simply the unwitting victims of a sordid political campaign against Chiropractic that has long been waged by that totally self-serving political powerhouse, the American Medical Association.

It is the AMA that vehemently opposes Chiropractic. And, its opposition has assumed the form of a carefully-planned, well-organized, all-out offensive effort.

WILL THE REAL AMA PLEASE STAND UP?

People frequently ask, "Why aren't chiropractors recognized?"

The best response to this question is another: "Recognized by whom?"

The answer, invariably, is, "The AMA."

Implicit in the initial question is the assumption that, in order for a system of health care to be valid, it would necessarily have to be approved by that organization. That is simply not true.

Wondering why chiropractors aren't recognized by the AMA is like wondering why Democrats aren't recognized by Republicans, or why Roman Catholics aren't recognized by Jews. In each example, the two factions involved simply represent opposing points of view on a common issue. It is widespread knowledge that, in such situations, the more threatening the opposing viewpoint, the greater the protestations that are voiced. This is especially true if the one doing the protesting is the reigning autocrat in a particular jurisdiction, which is precisely the case in this instance.

SO, WHERE'S THE BEEF?

Clearly, the average person thinks of the American Medical Association as the "watchdog" of health and health care, existing solely in the interest of public welfare. Equally clearly, most people probably think that the AMA represents all or nearly all of the medical profession.

Neither assumption is true. In fact, they are quite far off base. First of all, it might surprise you to know that approximately 58% of all medical doctors in the U.S. are AMA members. Almost half the profession has resigned or declined membership, largely because of disenchantment with the organization.

Secondly, although the AMA would certainly have you believe that it had your best interests as its first priority, it is actually far more concerned with its own well-being and that of its member doctors. The organization's motivation is not quite what one might think.

The AMA is the political arm of the medical profession. It is a *trade organization*, and as such, it is *bound by charter to protect its member MD's*. Far more important than your personal welfare is the AMA's monopolistic control of the health care system and the earning potential of its members. It sounds almost un-American to say this, but it is indeed the truth.

The AMA has opposed virtually every competing health care profession that has come along and posed a threat to Medicine's supremacy, including Podiatry, Osteopathy, Optometry and Dentistry. Although these professions eventually managed to slip through the cracks and take a foothold, in no case did it come easily. And, AMA efforts against these professions pale in comparison to it attack against Chiropractic.

The AMA has also gone on record as opposing practically all social legislation that served the interests of public welfare, such as Medicare, Medicaid, child labor laws, social security, minimum wage legislation, the 40-hour work week, and more. Why? Because it was somehow deemed in the best interest of the AMA to do so.

THE CONFUSION ABOUT CHIROPRACTORS

The American Medical Association boasts one of the richest and most powerful lobbies in Washington, spending more than $5 million in a typical election year in order to get its proponents into office. It has the power to manipulate and influence legislators almost at will. Interestingly, one of the bolder assertions in AMA anti-Chiropractic propaganda is that Chiropractic has only become legitimized because of its "intensive and amazingly skillful political campaigning." In light of its own political strength, it is ludicrous to believe that the AMA Goliath could have lost a purely political battle to the Chiropractic David. For Chiropractic to have won legislative support and federal, state and local sanction in the face of such overwhelming opposition indicates that evidence in its favor must have been undeniable.

Despite the phenomenal manipulative power and the vast influence of the AMA, its questionable tactics have not gone unnoticed. A number of legislators have voiced their disapproval of the organization and its strategies. Senator Edward M. Kennedy issued the following scathing remarks in a 1971 address to his subcommittee on administrative practices:

> . . . Instead of the scientific and public professional organization it was founded as, the AMA has turned into a propaganda organ purveying "medical politics," for deceiving the Congress, the people, and the doctors of America themselves. The American Medical Association puts the lives and well-being of American citizens below its own special interests in ordering its priorities. It deserves to be ignored, rejected, and forgotten.

Never has the AMA been so aggressive as it has in its attempt to — in its own words — "contain and eliminate the chiropractic menace." It has spared no amount of time, money or energy toward this end. In fact, it has been said that, in light of the social and ethical value of the legislation and other professions that the AMA has opposed, the Chiropractic profession should be especially flattered to be the object of such intense and single-minded hostility.

SO, WHERE'S THE BEEF?

THE COMMITTEE ON QUACKERY

The AMA efforts against Chiropractic all began in 1963, with the formation of the AMA *Committee on Quackery*. Established because AMA officials had become concerned that medical doctors were cooperating with chiropractors, the Committee developed the sole written objective of "directing its attention to the chiropractic problem," with the ultimate purpose being "the containment and elimination of Chiropractic."

Activities of the Committee included suppressing research favorable to Chiropractic, undermining Chiropractic colleges and postgraduate educational programs, making ethical rulings that prevented medical doctors from associating with chiropractors or Chiropractic colleges, and subverting a U.S. government inquiry into the merits of Chiropractic. In addition, it began a massive misinformation campaign against Chiropractic, carefully designed to totally discredit the profession and its practitioners. Using half-truths, innuendoes, obsolete information and isolated incidents of malpractice, and utilizing such inflammatory terms as "unscientific," "cultist," "untrained," and "rabid dogs," the AMA systematically planted seeds of doubt, mistrust and fear in the minds of the public, the fruits of which are now being enjoyed.

The Committee on Quackery took measures to thwart Chiropractic at every level. Its game plan included attempts to: "encourage chiropractic disunity," "encourage ethical complaints against chiropractors," and to "oppose chiropractic inroads in health insurance, . . . in workmen's compensation, . . . into labor unions, . . . and into hospitals." This policy of containment was expected to eventually cause the profession to "wither and die on the vine."

Although the AMA Committee on Quackery no longer exists, it has left an enduring signature in the form of Chiropractic's negative and spurious image. There isn't a chiropractor alive who doesn't encounter the fruits of the Committee's labor on a daily basis.

THE CONFUSION ABOUT CHIROPRACTORS

THE "CHICAGO FIVE"

Tired of suffering the indignities that went along with Chiropractic's negative public image, a group of five Illinois chiropractors filed a lawsuit in 1976, claiming unlawful conspiracy in restraint of trade on the part of the AMA and numerous associated organizations. The chiropractors sought damages for loss of reputation and income, in addition to injunctions forbidding any further such illegal activities.

After eleven long years and millions of dollars in expenses (in a battle against an opponent with almost unlimited available funds), the lawsuit was finally decided in favor of the chiropractors. The court found the American Medical Association *guilty* of illegally boycotting the Chiropractic profession. Evidence of the illegalities included documentation of the mission of the Committee on Quackery, proof of all the aforementioned anti-Chiropractic efforts, and documentation of American Hospital Association threats "to withdraw and refuse accreditation of a hospital that granted privileges to chiropractors." The court acknowledged that the latter denial would likely be a devastating factor to any hospital involved, very possibly leading to closure.

During the course of the trial, the lawyers for the AMA repeatedly attempted to introduce evidence that Chiropractic posed serious health hazards. The response of the court to such evidence was that it was "incredible and unworthy of belief."

The court enjoined the AMA and its affiliated organizations from any further illegal activities, and encouraged interprofessional association and cooperation. Additionally, citing that the AMA has "never acknowledged the lawlessness" of its "systematic wrongdoing and intent to destroy a licensed profession," the court ordered the AMA to send copies of the Order of Injunction to each of its 275,000 members, to publish it in the *Journal of the American Medical Association*, and to declare it ethical for a medical physician to associate professionally with chiropractors.

This landmark decision promises to benefit both the Chiropractic profession and the American public, and may one day help to bring Chiropractic the equality it deserves. But this won't happen overnight. Despite the fact that the AMA's tactics have been denounced as illegal, the truth is that those tactics have been extremely effective. Public sentiment is influenced residually to this day, and much of the damage that has been done to Chiropractic's reputation will be difficult to repair.

Regardless of the facts of the lawsuit, most medical doctors maintain their anti-Chiropractic persuasion, which necessarily influences their interactions with patients. There remains a strong climate of opposition to Chiropractic in medical schools, which will not vanish simply on the basis of a lawsuit. The reality of the situation is that interprofessional relations have not improved measurably, nor are they likely to in the near future.

With public and medical sentiment still decidedly anti-Chiropractic, the AMA's desired illusion remains intact. Chiropractic's struggle will be an arduous one as long as the AMA maintains its stronghold on the forces that influence public opinion.

THE AMA'S SPHERE OF INFLUENCE

Although its methods have been declared illicit, the American Medical Association still wields its mighty sword, particularly in the media, where its position on any issue is seemingly accepted without question as the last word.

Journalists and editors seem especially vulnerable to AMA influence. Newspaper and magazine articles about Chiropractic typically reek of AMA flavor. Of the few books that one can find that are either about Chiropractic or mention it in specific context, most hold it in a negative light. Some, in fact, have been sanctioned — and perhaps even paid for — by the AMA.

One must wonder why and how so many seemingly responsible journalists have fallen prey to AMA influence. One thing that is known is that Ann Landers — a frequent and often vicious critic of Chiropractic — has travelled to China at the expense of the American Medical Association. Since her opinion is regarded as gospel by millions of unsuspecting readers (she has even been referred to as "the most influential woman in the world"), her AMA-influenced views have undoubtedly been damaging to Chiropractic.

Another area in which the AMA aroma is evident is the *insurance* industry. Although the AMA was unsuccessful in its attempts to prevent "Chiropractic inroads" into health insurance, its influence is very noticeable in insurance procedures and attitudes.

Even though most health insurance policies include Chiropractic coverage (and, in fact, many states have passed "insurance equity" laws that supposedly guarantee equal coverage for chiropractic care), limits of coverage often appear arbitrary and subjective, based upon the interpretation of need rendered by individual "medical consultants" employed by insurance companies. In this author's personal experience, the typical medical consultant is neither particularly fond of, nor especially knowledgeable about, Chiropractic. With the limits of coverage arbitrarily set by people who know little and think less of Chiropractic, claims for payment are frequently unreasonably denied.

Denial is often based on the determination that services rendered are beyond that considered "reasonable and customary" for the particular condition, or that such services are not "medically necessary." Given the medical consultant's characteristic position on Chiropractic, the likelihood of his or her deeming chiropractic services to be medically necessary is about the same as the likelihood of a rabbi bringing home a pound of bacon.

Often patients are directed by their insurance companies to be evaluated by "independent medical examiners" in order to validate the need for chiropractic care. The examiners are usually medical orthopedists with anti-Chiropractic bias and no real understanding of how or why chiropractic treatment works. Although these qualities would seem to make them unqualified to evaluate the need for or efficacy of chiropractic care, they are put in the position of making such determinations. Not only do they usually recommend against any further chiropractic treatment, but many of these examiners have been known to discredit Chiropractic at every opportunity.

SO, WHERE'S THE BEEF?

All of the above are examples of subtle yet effective repression of the Chiropractic profession. As it is plain to see, the Committee on Quackery lives on, if only in spirit.

Every chiropractic physician sees clear evidence of AMA handiwork every time a patient expresses fear about telling his or her "regular" doctor about having seen the chiropractor. The fear, based on the illusion of the chiropractor as a marginal practitioner, is not without foundation: not uncommonly, patients bold enough to make the disclosure receive angry, indignant responses. Typical of such replies is this one, heard just the other day: "Why in the world you are seeing *him*? Don't you know those people can *hurt* you?"

AN UNSCIENTIFIC CULT

Early on in its war against Chiropractic, the American Medical Association began referring to its rival profession as an "unscientific cult." All of the AMA's anti-Chiropractic propaganda contained this derogatory term, and one can well imagine how effective it was in frightening off prospective patients. Coining the expression was, in fact, a stroke of genius: just the sound of it evokes images of ranting, raving lunatics dancing wildly around a fire clad in bizarre costumes.

The AMA has always claimed that chiropractic principles are not based upon the commonly accepted body of knowledge in the area of health and disease. The truth is quite the contrary. The principles of Chiropractic are supported and documented by valid medical literature and research findings, some of which have been mentioned previously. Spinal mechanical principles are known fact, not merely chiropractic hypothesis, and the basis for the work that chiropractors do is not "the chiropractic theory of health and disease," but rather the anatomy and physiology of the human body. Although much is still unknown about the body, there is mounting evidence in support of the chiropractic claim that removing nerve interference by correcting spinal subluxations can help to prevent and cure disease and prolong life. And certainly, the musculo-skeletal effects of spinal mechanical impairment require no further proof.

After all, what is a "science," anyway? Webster defines *science* as "the study and theoretical explanation of natural phenomena." By definition, Chiropractic is no less scientific than Medicine.

Clearly, health care is not an exact science. It is, one could say, more *art* than science. Considering the customary interpretation of the word "science," which infers *precision* and *certainty*, there seems little that is scientific about the practice of Medicine. In fact, it could well be said that the medical critics of Chiropractic live in the proverbial glass house. Many of the *drugs* commonly prescribed by medical doctors work by "unknown mechanisms of action." In other words, nobody has even a remote idea how they work, but we know what we can probably expect to happen. Doctors prescribe them freely, without really knowing what they do to the bodies of the people who take them. Even aspirin — the most basic of all medications — works by an unknown mechanism.

And, even in the case of drugs with *known* mechanisms of action, taking them may well do more harm than good. There is no such thing as a drug with no harmful side effects.

This author has a patient, a lovely 72-year-old lady whom we will call Glenda. Glenda suffers from moderate degenerative arthritis, occasional dizziness, chronic shoulder bursitis, chronic upper back pain caused by two healed compression fractures in her spine (which are common in elderly people and involve a compressing, or crushing, of the considerably-more-fragile vertebrae, with subsequent healing and relatively little functional disturbance), moderately elevated blood pressure, and what she describes as "occasional depression."

In treating her, Glenda's "regular" doctor has turned her into a walking chemistry laboratory. At last count, she was taking no fewer than 10 drugs on a regular basis, all of which were prescribed by the same physician. A brief look at her daily "menu" will be quite revealing:

(1) **Doxidan**. A laxative. Apparently, she suffers from occasional constipation. This drug is reasonably safe if taken only occasionally and according to directions.

(2) **Clinoril.** A member of the family of drugs known as "non-steroidal anti-inflammatory" medications, Clinoril relieves inflammation, pain and fever. It can also very effectively cause peptic ulcer, gastro-intestinal bleeding, inhibited blood clotting, liver malfunction, kidney toxicity, swelling in the legs, nausea, vomiting, constipation *or* diarrhea, dizziness, headache, nervousness, depression, and Congestive Heart Failure. *The mechanism of action is unknown.*

(3) **Quinamm.** This is what is known as a "neuromuscular agent." It relaxes muscle tissue. It can also cause a rash, fever, digestive upset, disturbed breathing, ringing in the ears, visual impairment, deafness, dizziness, headache, nausea, vomiting, confusion, and angina pectoris (heart-related chest pain).

(4) **Clonopin.** This is an "anti-convulsive." None of Glenda's symptoms seem to have warranted the use of this medication; she doesn't remember why it was prescribed for her, but one can only assume that the doctor had a logical reason. This drug produces depression (One of the recommendations for anyone on this drug is to "avoid any activities requiring mental alertness"). It may actually *increase* the incidence of seizures (One must wonder why this drug is on the market at all). It can also cause such side effects as spasticity, coma, slurred speech, headache, depressed respiration, confusion, hallucinations, insomnia, heart palpitations, hair loss *or* excessive hair growth, anorexia, enlarged liver, and blood abnormalities.

(5) **Fiorinal with Codeine.** This drug "raises the threshold of pain and discomfort." In other words, let the fire rage on, but turn off the alarm. Other potential adverse reactions are few in number, with the worst being nausea and vomiting.

(6) **Adapin.** Here again, its mechanism of action is unknown. What is known is that its predominant action is on the Central

Nervous System. This drug's effects are anti-anxiety, anti-depression, and anti-insomnia. Here is a particularly interesting possibility: it can "unmask latent psychotic symptoms." Additionally, it can cause rapid heartbeat, extremely low blood pressure, altered gait, digestive upset, fatigue, blurred vision, "pins and needles" sensations, and more.

(7) **Tenoretic.** This drug is used primarily for high blood pressure. It reduces heart rate, blood pressure, and cardiac output (which implies that anyone on this drug can only perform moderately active tasks). It can cause cardiac failure or heart attack, and is known to react negatively with Adapin (drug #6 on the menu). It can cause depression (to the point of being catatonic), hallucinations, disorientation, and what is politely termed a "slightly clouded sensorium" (translation: you may have only a vague idea of where you are and what you're doing).

(8) **Norpramin.** This is an anti-depressant whose mechanism of action is unknown. It, too, works on the Central Nervous System. In someone with cardiac disease, it can cause heart attack; it may encourage seizures, it blocks the action of blood pressure medication, interacts negatively with other anti-depressants, and can cause low *or* high blood pressure. Additionally, it can cause a rapid heartbeat, stroke, numbness, tingling, "pins and needles," lack of coordination, hallucinations, delusions, blood disorders, hormone disorders, and more.

(9) **Parafon Forte.** Its mode of action is unknown, but it *seems* to relieve symptoms like pain, stiffness, and limitation of motion. It relaxes muscle spasm. Concomitant use of Central Nervous System depressants may cause adverse reactions. This drug is described as being "well-tolerated, with mild side effects," which include possible gastrointestinal bleeding, drowsiness, lightheadedness, dizziness and liver damage.

(10) **Amitryptilene.** This is an anti-depressant and sedative with an unknown mechanism of action. Interaction with another anti-depressant can cause high fever, severe convulsions, or even death. This drug may block the action of blood pressure medication. It can also cause heart attack, stroke, high *or* low blood pressure, loss of coordination, hallucinations, hepatitis, and other serious symptoms.

These drugs are devastating! There isn't one on the list that ought to be taken under any but the most dire circumstances. Any one of them can cause problems far more serious than those it may help. Practically any of them can be potentially fatal; taking them in combination is Russian roulette.

Even though some of these drugs are known to interact negatively with each other, even though their cumulative effects are terribly dangerous, and even though Glenda probably doesn't need any of them, her "regular" doctor has placed her on all of them. If you were reading carefully, you probably noticed that many of Glenda's symptoms come right from the laundry list of side effects of her medications. Not only that, but several of the drugs are known to negate the actions of some of the others, rendering them even more useless than normal. And obviously, some of the medications have been prescribed to counter the side effects of others.

Glenda walks around in a constant daze, confused, disoriented, dizzy, lightheaded, and depressed. She suffers from insomnia, chest pains, ringing in her ears, frequent tingling and "pins and needles" sensations in her arms and legs, an erratic gait, and other symptoms that are suspiciously familiar to those of us who have read the preceding pages. It's painfully clear that these symptoms have all been drug-induced, as a result of what appears an almost criminal abuse of medical license.

If Glenda were to die tomorrow, or next week, or next month, from a heart attack, stroke, or perhaps liver failure, how do you suppose people — including her physician — would perceive her death? They would say that *she was 72 years old, and her health had been gradually deteriorating. She died of natural causes.* Hogwash! The cause of her death would be physician-induced drug abuse. Offhand, one could say that Medicine was an unscientific cult.

UNTRAINED?

In much of the AMA-generated literature, the comment has been made that chiropractors are inadequately trained to diagnose and treat human illness. Obsolete and erroneous information is used as evidence in support of this claim. Based on the facts, it is obvious that chiropractors are well-qualified to render health care. There is, however, an important distinction to point out here, involving the process known as *diagnosis.* Diagnosis is the identification of disease by careful analysis and examination. The statement that chiropractors are untrained and unqualified to diagnose implies that medical doctors are eminently competent diagnosticians. This is not the case at all.

According to a number of reliable authorities, *the best diagnosticians are correct in their diagnoses one-third of the time.* And, if those statistics represent the very best in diagnostic acumen, it means that the *average* among health care professionals is probably 20 or 25 percent. So, it's time to call a spade a spade; diagnosis doesn't really exist. At best, it is educated guesswork.

Based on those facts alone, it is apparent that you shouldn't take a medication of any kind unless there is no viable alternative. According to the statistics, you would probably be taking the drug on the basis of a mistaken diagnosis. Taken for a condition that has been diagnosed correctly, drugs are destructive enough; what rational person would take one knowing the truth about diagnostic statistics? For that matter, what rational person would *prescribe* one knowing these facts?

Chiropractic works. It isn't the answer for all health problems, because there is no one answer. But it effectively treats many different conditions without drugs or surgery and, unlike those methods, there is little chance of harmful side effects or irrevocable harm. To deny the obvious benefits of this system of health care is ludicrous.

SO, WHERE'S THE BEEF?

What does the American Medical Association stand to gain by continuing to oppose Chiropractic? It's quite simple, really. It gets to eliminate very viable competition in the marketplace, thereby maintaining a virtual monopoly of the health care system. And, it gets to continue its autocratic control over all health-related issues.

How is the public affected by all of this? Because of their mistaken notions about Chiropractic, millions of people refrain from seeking chiropractic care for disabling and painful problems that could be effectively treated and corrected. Instead, they "go to the doctor" and receive inappropriate and ineffective care. Moreover, our untreated spinal fixations and subluxations are silently paving the way for future serious health problems. And, we continue to be a "crisis medicine"-oriented society, passively and resolutely awaiting our fate, instead of a "wellness"-oriented one, actively controlling our own destinies.

8

Ignorance: Who Pays the Price?

Being a chiropractor can be extremely frustrating. To know just how much you are able to help people, and yet to know that relatively few people know that, is very difficult to deal with. There are almost daily reminders of how little people know about what you do, and how little people generally regard it.

I frequently run into people who have been patients at my office and who, in fact, have achieved wonderful results from my treatment. In some cases, the response was nothing short of miraculous, often in chronic conditions of years' duration. It amazes me to hear what these people sometimes have to say.

CHARLOTTE

One woman, whom I will call Charlotte, had come to me complaining of headaches that she had been having for over twenty years. These were not just headaches; they were HEADACHES — constant, non-stop, morning-to-night, twenty-year-old headaches. She had been to numerous other physicians over the years — all of whom had concurred with the diagnosis of chronic migraine headaches — and had only been able to obtain occasional, temporary relief from her discomfort with various medications. Much of her time was spent in a "fog" created by one or another of these drugs. (We must keep reminding ourselves that this is known as "health care.") Charlotte's headaches were simply a part of her daily routine.

In situations like this one, much of the chiropractor's work has already been done for him by the time the patient enters the office. Charlotte had had CAT scans, brain scans, skull X-rays and the entire gamut of laboratory tests, along with extensive medical examinations, none of which had turned up anything "serious." No tumors, blood clots, inflammatory conditions of the brain or spinal cord, nothing. Nothing serious: only 20 years of blinding, debilitating, torturous headaches. The poor woman had been around the block and back, with virtually no success at all. Literally everything else had been ruled out but mechanical spinal involvement. In fact, spinal involvement had never been considered as a possibility by the "real doctors" Charlotte had consulted. In cases like this, chiropractic care is almost always successful at getting rid of the problem, or at least providing far more relief than has been previously obtained.

Predictably, my examination revealed that Charlotte had spinal fixations that typically demonstrate a high degree of correlation with headaches, and I told her so. I explained that I felt confident that we had an excellent chance of correcting her problem, but that it was certainly a chronic, stubborn problem that was going to require a good deal of work: months, in fact, to successfully mobilize the locked-up spinal joints that were most likely causing her headaches. Of course, she happily agreed to begin treatment.

After about two months of treatments, Charlotte's headaches were completely gone. They had vanished without a trace! Mind you, this is after 20 years of her being a headache with legs, and after every medical attempt to help her had failed. (A typical M.D.'s reaction: "A coincidence. The headaches were 'self-limiting'; they would have gone away on their own.")

Charlotte was, needless to say, beside herself. And me? I was a hero. Talk about gratification!

As I had been very careful to explain, it was important that she continue with her treatments. Although her headaches were gone, I could see that the underlying spinal impairment was not yet totally corrected. After all, I reasoned, our objective was not just to relieve her pain, although that was a fabulous result; our ultimate goal was to correct the cause of the problem so that the headaches didn't return.

Nothing I could say was able to overcome a lifetime of medical orientation. Charlotte stopped coming in for care as soon as she felt better. Almost always, when a patient stops treatment that way, the symptoms eventually return, and I made sure to tell her so.

"Oh, if they do," she said, "you can be sure that I'll be back in for treatment." After twenty years of having a headache for a constant companion, she was unwilling to follow my recommendations for continuing the treatment program to its very logical conclusion. I could only shake my head.

When I eventually ran into Charlotte on the street, it had been almost a full year since I had last seen her in my office. Soon enough, I got around to asking her about her headaches. Her response floored me.

"Oh," she said, "they came back after about three months. It got so bad that I went to the headache clinic down in Greenwich. They put me on an experimental drug that seems to be working pretty well. As long as I stay on it, the headaches are tolerable. Sometimes, I don't even notice them. The medicine makes me a little groggy, though, and sometimes upsets my stomach."

The joy of Chiropractic!

NED

Another patient had come to me with troublesome neck pain and stiffness that had been bothering him for several months. After the appropriate examination procedures, I presented my findings, which correlated quite well with his symptoms. I told him that in order to be effective, I had to see him approximately three times per week for probably four or five weeks, and then perhaps for additional treatments with diminishing frequency.

Ned was very frank with me. "Doc," he said, "I'm a terrible patient. I can guarantee you that I'll stop coming in as soon as I feel better."

I think a doctor should appreciate that kind of candor from a patient; at least it tells you where you stand. But I had to tell Ned that if he chose to handle it that way — which was indeed his prerogative — he could probably count on the symptoms returning after a while. He understood, and assured me (as Charlotte had) that he would return for treatment in the event that should happen. We set about the task of handling his problem.

Ned was free from pain after about three weeks of care, and we parted amicably. That was over a year ago.

He recently stopped by the office, and I overheard him telling my office manager the reason he came in. It was to pick up his X-rays so that he could take them to an orthopedic surgeon.

Upon hearing that, I asked if he had been in an accident or suffered an injury in some other way. No, he assured me, he was just feeling the same old pain again in his neck. He said it had been fine for about six months, but that he had then begun to develop a vague discomfort that had recently begun to bother him sufficiently to prompt him to do something about it.

"Ned," I said, "why don't you just get started with treatments again, and this time let me correct the problem fully, before it's no longer correctable?"

His response was predictable if exasperating: "Well, maybe I will, but first I want to see what a *regular* doctor has to say about it."

ESTHER

Most frustrating of all are the patients who could more accurately call *im*patients. Typical of this type person was Esther, a woman who came to see me after having suffered with neck and arm pain for many months, and having been told by her neurosurgeon that she absolutely needed surgery.

After doing my usual workup for such conditions, I described to her what I felt was causing her problem. We discussed fixations, subluxations, nerve interference, and so on, and I expressed optimism that the problem might respond to chiropractic management, obviating the need for surgery. Of course, she was elated to even think that there might be that chance.

I was very careful to explain that the treatment regimen was going to have to be quite intensive, involving several treatments per week for a number of weeks. I told her not to expect rapid relief from her symptoms, since her problem was a chronic one that required a great deal of care, and there are just no magic wands in chiropractic treatment. Esther assured me that she understood, and again told me how grateful she was that I had given her a measure of hope. I had every reason to believe that I was dealing with a patient who understood the situation, who knew the nature of our objectives, and who would follow my recommendations to a T.

I began treating her and, although I had been right about her not experiencing immediate relief, I was pleased with what I felt was definite mechanical improvement after just four or five treatments.

You can imagine my surprise, then, when I received a message that she had cancelled her next appointment and did not intend to return. Naturally, I called her at home to find out if there was some problem. Her explanation was that *she just didn't feel any better*, and so she wasn't coming back. No amount of reminding her about our earlier conversations was able to get her to reconsider. She just wasn't coming back, and that was all there was to it. Apparently, she had decided that surgical dismemberment of her spine was a more appealing alternative.

Chances are that somebody "got to her." Some well-intentioned person — her surgeon, a relative, a friend — probably said something to her, like, "What on earth are you going to *one of them* for? Don't you know that those quacks can hurt you?"

GOOD OLD DOC SMITH

Among the most exasperating patients to deal with are those who expect me to do exactly what was done for them previously by someone else, either a chiropractor or an osteopath (some of whom work quite a bit like chiropractors). Usually these patients are older, and their other doctors have either retired or passed away. The conversation usually goes something like this:

"I know exactly what I need. Old Doc Smith — he's dead now — used to put me on my side and just crack my back, right here (pointing to a spot), and I'd get up feeling like a million bucks."

"Tell me," I say, "how long ago was that?"

"Oh, I'd say about twenty years ago. But I'm sure this is the same thing. All you have to do is crack me right here (pointing again)."

These patients invariably go on to tell me that they want no examination, no X-rays, nothing but a good, old-fashioned "back crackin'."

Of course, a responsible doctor of Chiropractic will never do that. At the very least, it is necessary to perform the minimal examination procedure that will give the doctor a reasonable understanding of the nature of the problem. Treating a person in the way he or she prescribes based upon something that occurred 20 years ago is like reading a newspaper that is 20 years old and living your life as though the news in it were current.

Sometimes these patients agree to an examination, and sometimes they don't. If not, I cordially suggest that they try another office.

But even if they do relent, these situations rarely prove satisfying to either doctor or patient. They are like two rams butting heads. The patient may follow the doctor's recommendations, but does so totally against his will. No matter how the doctor tries to explain it to him, he simply won't understand that that was then, and this is now. Joints change, muscles change, the body ages, and treatment and examination procedures change. And, I'm not good old Doc Smith (who could, by the way, walk on water). These situations rarely go well. A patient such as this has unrealistic expectations and will usually disappear after two or three treatments, convinced that I couldn't shine Doc Smith's shoes.

And so, even people who are somehow able to overcome their AMA-inspired fears enough to seek chiropractic care are often unable to derive the full benefit of their treatment, simply because of their medical orientation. As a chiropractor, one soon learns to appreciate the perseverance of salmon, who must forever swim against the current.

9 Innate Intelligence

INNATE INTELLIGENCE

Critics of Chiropractic seem to enjoy ridiculing the Chiropractic reverence for what the profession calls "Innate Intelligence." This is simply another attempt to defile a perfectly reasonable tenet.

Innate Intelligence — often simply referred to as "Innate" by chiropractors — is the term that has always been used within the profession in reference to the human body's own inherent ability to regulate itself. The remarkable *life force* possessed by the body, the body's ability to heal its own wounds and mend its broken bones — indeed, the very *wisdom* shown by the body as it methodically supervises its myriad activities — this is what chiropractors mean by the term Innate Intelligence.

There is no question that a life force exists in the body. While each of us goes merrily about our business, our bodies quietly manage all of the biological functions necessary for us to do so. The heart beats, the lungs breathe, the stomach and intestines digest, the kidneys and liver filter and detoxify, and so on, all without our own conscious control. The body instinctively knows to carry out these functions, and is equipped with the computer-like ability to do so on its own. It is truly amazing.

The medical community does acknowledge this phenomenon, but, as might be expected, it does so almost begrudgingly. In referring to the life force that directs the body's activities, the medical preference is to use the term

127

homeostasis, which means "balance," or "equilibrium" (as in, the normal state of the body when all functions are in order). And so, in typical medical understatement, the concession is made that the body does indeed have something to do with running its own activities.

Never mind that the body somehow *knows* to heal a cut when it occurs, or to mend a broken bone. *Never mind* that it handles the various physiological functions mentioned above on its own, continuously, and usually flawlessly. *Never mind* that 100 trillion specialized cells are constantly carrying out their individual functions in a beautifully orchestrated effort, and reproducing themselves identically when they somehow know that their useful lives have been used up, so that succeeding generations of cells can carry on family tradition. *Never mind* that Man never has and never will be able to duplicate human life. *Never mind all that*; the body simply regulates itself, that's all.

Many doctors have the self-centered notion that they heal people. It's not true. No doctor heals anybody; the body heals itself. The best a doctor can hope to do is create the most effective environment for healing to occur.

The body's self-regulatory powers, its recuperative abilities, the very miracle of Life — yes, I would call that Wisdom. I'd call it a Life Force. I'd even call it Innate Intelligence. Certainly, it's a great deal more than "homeostasis."

Those that criticize the chiropractor's reverence for the body's Innate Intelligence make the statement that Innate is considered to be a "God-given force that flows through the body." Taken out of context, this would seem consistent with the "unscientific cult" theme. You can begin to see the kind of mileage that has been gotten out of that image.

Hippocrates, the acknowledged "Father of Medicine," spoke about the existence of a life force. He called it the *vis medicatrix naturae* (the Latin term for "healing force of nature"). The eastern cultures refer to it as *ch'i* (which means, literally, "life force"), and hold it in the highest esteem.

We all know that a rose by any name would smell as sweet. Call it what you will, Innate Intelligence not only exists, but is the compelling force of life.

This discussion underscores the basis of Chiropractic and of wholistic health care. The human body is an intricate system with many integrated component parts. To treat it as a collection of disconnected, segregated, independent pieces — as is most often done in conventional medical practice — makes no sense. Where is the logic in treating a *shoulder*, or a *back*, or a *head*, or a *stomach*? What's sensible about viewing a person as a headache, an ulcer, or a kidney stone?

And yet, doctors tend to talk in those terms. A fly on the wall of a room full of MD's would hear remarks like the following:

"I had a really interesting neuralgia today."

"I had a hot low back come in today."

"I've got to operate on a disc in the morning."

"I had a real tough shoulder this afternoon."

"I saw a classic migraine the other day."

"I've got a knee at nine and a shoulder at noon."

What an insult to Humankind! Our health care system has reduced us to a collection of symptoms and assorted body parts, totally losing sight of the miracle of Life in the process.

The problem with too many doctors is that they have such little regard for the body's life force that they feel that they can and should control it. Such wanton disregard for the integrity of the human body is at the core of the failure of our system of health care to adequately serve our needs.

But the blame doesn't rest only on the shoulders of health providers. We, the people, have bought their line. We live in a society in which the Almighty Doctor is worshipped as a god.

Bernie Siegel, M.D. (author of the wonderful book, *LOVE, MEDICINE, AND MIRACLES*) is one medical doctor who has not lost sight of the Miracle of Life, and his exceptional results in the treatment of "terminally ill" patients reflects his love and respect for people and for the human body. He states his suspicion that the initials *M.D.* stand for "Medical Deity."

Perhaps we should abandon the practice of worshipping doctors, and develop a cultural reverence for the Miracle of the Human Body. Such a reverence would practically compel us to live a "wellness" lifestyle that would enable us to live longer and better lives. It would also demand a system of health care that was based on maintaining and enhancing well-being and preventing disease.

Such a system already exists. It is called Chiropractic.

* *

As usual, there was a long line outside the Pearly Gates, and the crowd of souls anxiously awaiting entrance into Heaven was growing restless.

As the nattering of the crowd grew louder, an elderly gent with a long, flowing white beard approached from the rear of the line. He was wearing a white lab coat and had a stethoscope hanging from his neck. The crowd watched in amazement as he approached the Gates and brazenly swaggered in past St. Peter, who passively allowed the line-crasher to enter.

"Hey!" shouted one of the more vocal members of the crowd, whose anger clearly spoke for the majority. "Who the heck does that guy think he is, jumping ahead of us that way?"

"Oh," St. Peter replied, "that's just God. He likes to play doctor."

10 The Proof of the Pudding

Arguments to the contrary aside, Chiropractic works. And it is often effective after all other methods have failed, which is arguably the most satisfying part of being a chiropractor. Chiropractic's track record could hardly be termed "coincidental."

The proof of the pudding is, as they say, in the eating. Every chiropractic physician has plenty of examples of the effectiveness of this method of treatment. What follows are a few case histories from my own files.

BOB C.

Bob C., a 38-year-old construction worker, came to my office complaining of low back pain that radiated into his right leg, hip and groin. He had been suffering from this condition for five months, during which time it had increased steadily in severity. By the time he came into the office, he was unable to sit at all. He couldn't work or get around very well. He was in constant misery. He was being maintained on pain-killing and muscle-relaxing medications, which were causing headaches, nausea, and other unpleasant side effects.

Five years earlier, Bob had had surgery to remove a ruptured disc in his low back. By the time he came to see me,

133

his doctor had told him that he needed to have another one removed. That was when a friend referred him to me.

A very real danger of disc surgery is that it severely compromises the mechanical function of the back, to the extent that adjacent discs can be worn down and damaged as a result of compensation. The surgically-repaired joint loses most of its mobility, and compensation in adjacent joints produces fixation, disc degeneration, and the danger of disc rupture at those levels. In a case like Bob's, that is always a consideration.

My examination led me to believe that I had a good chance of helping Bob, and I told him so. He didn't want another operation, so he was happy to follow my recommendation for several treatments a week.

Six weeks later, Bob was totally free from pain. His condition, however, required further treatment. I saw him weekly for approximately another six weeks, and eventually spread his visits to once every six weeks. With little exception, he has been coming for treatments on that basis over the past five years. Not only has he had no recurrence of his problem, but, in his words, the maintenance treatments have made him feel "ten years younger" than when he first came to see me.

There isn't a shred of doubt in my mind that Bob would have undergone back surgery for a second time if he hadn't come to see me, which would have only further compromised the function of his back and led to a lifetime of misery.

He recently told me, "Doc, you've given me a new life. You know, I hope you never move away, because if you do, it will mean that I'll have to sell my house and move with you."

JEANNE C.

Jeanne C. first came to my office as an admitted 45-year-old "nervous wreck." She suffered from a variety of symptoms, the worst of which was constant, chronic low back pain. She had been to many doctors before me, all of whom had told her that she had arthritis, and would have to "learn to live with it." The various medications she was taking were no doubt responsible for her nervousness, and they weren't doing much to help her so-called arthritis. When she came to me, she flatly told me that I was her last resort, and that her expectations weren't very high.

I performed the usual thorough examination, which included X-rays and laboratory tests. Interestingly, there was no evidence of arthritis of any kind. There was, however, a tremendous amount of spinal fixation and imbalance. There was also evidence that her adrenal glands — the organs in the body that help us cope with stress — were extremely sluggish. I treated her with a combination of spinal adjustments, physiotherapy, and nutritional supplementation. Two months later, all of her complaints were gone. She had no pain, needed no medication, and was as calm and cool as a person can be. Now, several years later, I still see her for maintenance care about every six weeks.

As some patients are prone to do, Jeanne wrote me a letter to express her gratitude. Here is what she said:

Dear Dr. DeRoeck,

It is very difficult for me to express how I feel now, as I'm not one to use adjectives very much, and since the whole thing is like a miracle, I tend to go overboard.

But, here it goes:

Truly, it seems impossible to believe the total effect of my visits to your office. Before, because of all the pain I was constantly in, I became very quiet and introverted. All I could do at work would be to concentrate on getting through the day. Now I have no pain, do everything and I mean everything, including mowing the lawn, working in the garden, and teaching my 12-year-old how to play baseball; just everything I haven't been able to do for five years. Everyone at work and all my friends can't get over the change in me, and I think it's just fantastic.

One more thing: for six years I've been plagued with high blood pressure. The last time I went for a checkup, the nurse took my pressure, looked at me, and took it again. When the doctor came in, he took it. They couldn't believe how good it was. I feel this is another fringe benefit of my visits to your office.

Thank you,

Jeanne

BARBARA O.

Barbara O., an attractive 32-year-old woman, entered my office complaining of headaches and neck stiffness of four years' duration. She had been to other doctors for this, having been put on "all kinds of medication" for it, with poor results. She was referred to me by a friend who described her, symptomatically, as a "carbon copy" of herself, and whose problem had responded well to my treatments. My examination convinced me that Barbara's was in all probability a "chiropractic case," and I began treating her.

Within two weeks, her headaches were gone. As luck would have it, though, she was then involved in an automobile accident in which her car was struck from behind. The end result was a "whiplash" injury and a return of her headache and neck discomfort. Four more weeks of regular care were once again able to bring her total relief. The interval between treatments was gradually increased to about two months, and she continued to come in on that basis until she moved away a year later.

Before she left, Barbara thanked me for returning her to a "normal life," and for relieving her of the necessity of living on "all types of pills" to mask her pain.

ANN R.

Ann R., a 43-year-old woman experiencing the stress of being in the throes of a divorce, came to me complaining of pain and stiffness in her neck, with radiating numbness, pain and weakness into her left arm. It had first developed about three weeks previously, with no apparent provocation. She had been told by a medical doctor that she had a "pinched nerve," and was given anti-inflammatory, pain-killing, and tranquilizing medications to ease her discomfort. It was becoming progressively worse — not to mention the drugs' unpleasant side effects — and there was talk of surgery.

An extremely frank and direct person, Ann told me right off what I was up against. "Look," she said, "I have to tell you this. My father is a medical doctor, and he hates chiropractors. He thinks you're all quacks. But I don't want surgery, and I've heard so many good things about you in particular from so many of my friends. So, here I am."

After a thorough evaluation, which definitely revealed substantial spinal fixation, muscle spasm, and structural imbalance, I began treating her on the basis of three times per week. It took approximately two months, but we achieved total resolution of her problem. Now, a year after her initial visit, I see her about once every three or four weeks, primarily to help offset the physical effects of the stress in her life. Aside from the tension produced by her circumstances, she has experienced no return of her original symptoms.

"My only complaint," she says, "is that my father still refuses to talk about it."

THOMAS H.

When Thomas H.'s mother first brought him to see me, he was 2-1/2 years old. Practically since birth, he had suffered from a series of "colds," complicated by chest congestion and wheezing. At the time I first saw Thomas, these episodes were occurring approximately once a month, and would last for up to a week. He had been hospitalized once with pneumonia, and his chronic condition had been diagnosed as "asthmatic-type bronchial constriction." He had been on medication that included antibiotics and bronchial dilators.

My examination of Thomas told me that he did have spinal fixations in the upper back region, which is associated with the spinal nerve contribution to the lungs. I explained to his parents, both patients of mine, that although I couldn't be absolutely certain, I thought there was a good chance that Thomas would respond well to care. In any event, it couldn't hurt, and children normally respond very quickly, so we would know within a short time how effective my treatments were going to be.

I saw him once a week for a month, during which time his symptoms disappeared. Since the symptoms had always been of the variety that would come and go, I monitored his condition very carefully over the next few months, treating him every two weeks during that span. That took us through the winter, the first such season he had ever gotten through with no trace of colds or bronchial conditions of any kind. Interestingly, every preschool classmate had caught a cold or the flu at least once during that same period.

After the winter season, I spread out his treatments, first to one month, then to two, and finally to three months. I saw him quarterly for another year. Thomas is now ten years old. At this point, I see him once or twice a year. He has had no recurrence of his bronchial condition.

RICHARD D.

Richard D. was 33 years old when I first met him. He came to me with the specific complaint of low back and radiating leg pain that had developed after jogging several weeks earlier. He mentioned a history of back pain over a three-year period, characterized by recurring bouts of increasing severity.

A highly driven and successful businessman, Richard had a schedule that was very demanding, and he had a myriad of complaints that were less severe than his back pain, but which frequently made it difficult for him to function effectively.

My examination revealed an apparent spinal disc involvement that I felt could be helped by spinal adjustments. A six-week program of intensive treatments produced an excellent response. Not only was his back and leg pain gone, but he told me that he felt better than he ever had in his life.

"Before I began coming to the office," he said, "I had felt physically tired over a long period of time. And now , as a result of my treatments and the vitamins that you recommended, I am full of energy. In addition to that, not only is my low back and leg pain gone, but pains in my upper back and headaches that I was having are gone as well. And, my sinuses are even cured, after I had gone to a specialist with no results."

In a testimonial he asked to write for my office newsletter, he added:

"I would like to recommend that everybody who is considering a physical examination be sure to begin or end with a chiropractor."

JOHN L.

John L. didn't come to me initially as a patient. I had met him as a result of our mutual involvement in community theater, and we had become friends after having been involved in two shows together.

John was a bowler, and began experiencing severe discomfort in his hand and wrist to the point where it was interfering with his game and with his life in general. When he told me about it, I immediately suspected an involvement of the wrist known as *carpal tunnel syndrome.*

A thirty-second examination confirmed my suspicions. Since his condition was giving him so much trouble at that moment, I told him that I wanted to treat him right then and there.

Carpal tunnel syndrome frequently responds very well to a particular adjustment of the wrist that can easily be performed anywhere by one experienced in the technique. I adjusted John's wrist and he felt immediate relief that lasted the entire evening.

I had to repeat the adjustment twice more in the next two weeks before the condition appeared totally corrected. As I write this, it has been five months since that time, and John has experienced no further pain.

GAIL B.

Gail B. is a 39-year-old woman who came into my office complaining of pain in the region of her right shoulder blade that radiated into her armpit. The problem, she said, had developed about two months previously with no provocation, and was getting worse. She related a history of a ruptured disc in her neck that had occurred two years earlier and had responded reasonably well to cortisone injections. She also said that her medical doctor had recently given her a non-steroidal anti-inflammatory medication for her condition, and mentioned that surgery might ultimately be necessary to remove the damaged disc material.

I was able to view her CAT scan pictures, and saw that there was indeed a severely damaged disc in her neck. But my examination also revealed a great deal of mechanical impairment of surrounding joints as well, and I suspected that this might be the actual cause of her current symptoms. I told her that, but I also informed her that we couldn't be certain at all about the possible effectiveness of treatment. She decided that it would be worth pursuing, and we embarked on a program of care.

Gail's condition was a stubborn one, but she began to notice improvement after a month of care. After another month, her symptoms were greatly diminished and I was seeing a substantial change in the functional dynamics of her spine. We reduced the frequency of her visits to twice weekly, and after another month, to just once a week. By this time,

Gail's pain was completely gone, and she could turn her neck farther than she had been able to in years.

It has now been eight months since her initial visit, and she comes in once every month for maintenance care. There is little question that Gail would eventually have undergone surgery if she hadn't received chiropractic care, and that she would have been consigned to a life of chronic neck pain and misery. Instead, however, she can do anything she pleases, and is not only pain-free, but feels better than she has in years.

As the Epilogue to an old TV show used to say, "there are eight million stories (in the Naked City). This was only one of them." Every chiropractor who has been in practice for any length of time has hundreds of case histories just like those you have just read, stories that validate over and over the effectiveness of chiropractic health care.

Over the course of a number of years of practice, there is a tendency to take stories like these for granted, since such results are obtained daily in chiropractic offices. To the chiropractor, these cases are quite routine.

In truth, though, there is nothing routine about them. This is especially so when put into the perspective of the nature of health care in general and the prevailing attitude about Chiropractic. When seen in this light, results like those I have chronicled are nothing short of astounding.

What astounds *me,* when I consider how chiropractors routinely produce results of this nature, is the fact that the medical community continues to deny Chiropractic's effectiveness, and the general public continues to buy that malarkey. *That's* what astounds me!

11

Reflections About Life, Health, and Health Care

During the course of reading this book, you have undoubtedly been drawing your own conclusions about what you have been reading. By now you have an impression of Chiropractic that is probably quite different from the one you had before, or at least more complete. It is quite likely that you have also begun to look differently at some things you've been taking for granted up to now, namely the American Medical Association and our entire system of health care.

That's good. And, it's healthy. Not only is it both good and healthy, but it was precisely my purpose in writing this book.

I, too, have come to my own conclusions based on my years of experience as a chiropractic physician. During that time, I have come face to face with the far-reaching effects of the AMA's campaign against Chiropractic, and public misconception has been fired at me point blank. I have also had the opportunity to witness firsthand just what chiropractic treatment can do for people, and what it cannot do. I would like to share some of these observations with you.

First of all, it is clear to me that our entire system of health care needs restructuring. Its priorities are wrong, and it therefore does not serve us nearly as well as it ought to. As remarkable as some of its accomplishments are, our health care system betrays us.

Any system that legitimizes making laboratory rats out of innocent people like my patient, Glenda, and at the same time summarily discredits an amazingly effective, conservative, wellness-oriented method of treatment like Chiropractic, is badly missing the mark. Any system that treats the disease that has the person rather than the person that has the disease is falling far short of its responsibility. Any system that emphasizes cures more than prevention, and symptoms more than people, is missing the boat. Any system that permits a self-serving political organization like the AMA to wantonly disregard the rights and well-being of people in the pursuit of its own omnipotence is pathetically misdirected. And, any health care system that disregards vitally important, scientifically valid principles of health for reasons that are totally political is a miserable failure.

Chiropractic health care absolutely should be an integral part of the health care system. The spinal subluxation and the spinal fixation are critical factors in disease causation, and are as common as germs. Their importance should be recognized throughout all of health care and all of our society.

Not only should Chiropractic be a part of mainstream health care, but it should be an important part of each and every individual's personal program of health care and maintenance. Having your spinal subluxations and fixations detected and corrected ought to be as routine as having your teeth checked and cleaned by the dentist, working out at the health club, and having your annual physical. I firmly believe that anyone who understands the nature of spinal subluxations and fixations would be terribly foolish to not take the proper measures to ward them off. And, the one thing that must be remembered is that most of us are walking around with several such spinal impairments, which are interfering with our body mechanics, undermining our physical performance and health, setting the stage for disease, and very possibly shortening our lives. Moreover, this is all being permitted to occur because of medical politics.

There is an interesting development taking place. Although the AMA has long held its position that spinal manipulation is of no value, and that the principles of Chiropractic are unfounded, we are beginning to see the subtle emergence of both in the medical world, in what might very well be yet another carefully orchestrated effort to supplant Chiropractic.

There are two facets to this effort. First of all, there is a relatively new medical specialty known as *physiatry*. Physiatrists are described as being "doctors of physical medicine." They place emphasis on body mechanics, joint function, and structural balance, in a conservative approach to orthopedic problems. It would certainly appear from this description that the physiatrist is in reality a "medical chiropractor."

Secondly, *physical therapists* are now receiving specialized training in "spinal mobilization," and have begun to advertise this service. Since physical therapists function primarily by medical prescription, this represents another way in which the services of a chiropractor can be duplicated. Based upon the AMA's track record, one could easily imagine how this developing trend might have been masterminded by people within that organization. We can expect the day when the American Medical Association lays claim to the "discovery" of this extremely efficacious form of treatment, followed by the assertion that only physiatrists and physical therapists that have been "medically trained" are qualified to perform this highly specialized procedure.

Don't you believe that. No other health professional has anywhere near the calibre of training in the dynamics or manipulation of the spine that the chiropractor does, and it is safe to say that none ever will. Physiatrists pay the spine little heed, and the physical therapist's training in spinal mobilization is all too brief and sketchy. Even orthopedic surgeons and neurosurgeons have little appreciation for this marvel of natural architecture, nor do they understand how to prevent or resolve its mechanical problems. Only the chiropractor understands these things.

Chiropractors have a meaningful relationship with the human spine. The spine is very much the foremost object of the chiropractor's affection and attention, both during the educational experience and throughout professional practice. The spine is the chiropractor's heritage; it is his legacy. It is what every chiropractic physician knows best, and no one will ever know it quite as well.

No matter which or how many other health professionals begin to perform spinal manipulation, no matter who else undergoes specialized study of the spine, they will only be paying it lip service. They will only be giving it a cursory look, and regarding it as only of minor significance. It is very unlikely that the medical community will experience a major shift in the importance it attaches to spinal function; health care in general has strayed too far from Hippocrates' admonition to "look first to the spine." The AMA's sanctioning of courses in spinal manipulation is merely "covering all the bases." It is keeping pace with the Jones's. It will never do justice to the vital role of the spine in health and disease.

There is and always will be an important place on the health care team for the chiropractor. Not only that, but his or her place is right up on the front line. Chiropractic works, time and time again. Its effectiveness has been well-documented by years of clinical success and millions of happy and satisfied patients. It is no longer either appropriate or acceptable to disregard the value and importance of the Chiropractic paradigm of health care.

Health care must become much more than it is now. There will certainly always be a need for dedicated, talented practitioners of crisis medicine. They will always have an important role to play in health care, but it should be a *secondary* role. They should be called to action when natural, wholistic, preventive health care efforts have failed.

There are certain facts that we need to face. Not everyone will assume responsibility for doing all the right things for their optimal health. Being responsible for their health is not a high priority for some people, and they will always need to rely on crisis medicine to keep them going. But this should not be the central focus of health care, as it is today. Our only chance, as a society, to achieve improved health, increased longevity, and victory over the killer diseases of our culture, is to develop a health care system in which the best minds from all the health care disciplines work together in a united effort founded upon natural, wholistic, preventive principles. Our only hope is to teach people to assume control over all the factors that cause disease in the first place, and devote the lion's share of our time and energy to assisting people in attaining optimal health. Such an approach is infinitely more sensible than the current one of waiting for diseases to develop and then combatting them with drugs.

Health care should be about health instead of disease. It should be about being as well as you can be, and not just free of symptoms for the moment. It should be about "how healthy can I become?" instead of "oh, good, I don't have any symptoms today." It should be about prevention rather than cure, and about having sufficient vitality to run in road races at age 85, rather than being frail, sickly and debilitated (or *dead*). Health care should be about *actually dying of old age* — at 100 or older — instead of from a disease induced and nurtured by the very system that professes to be interested in our health. And finally, health care should be a cooperative effort of dedicated physicians from all health disciplines, rather than a political prize fight in which the championship belt is *the marketplace*. You deserve so much more than you're getting.

I believe that if we actually had a health care system that emphasized the principles of health — nutrition, exercise, stress control, proper health habits, and structural integrity — we would be able to reduce disease by more than 50%, and increase the average lifespan to at least 85 years. We've gotten so far away from the real principles of health and disease — as a result of our infatuation with revolutionary cures and treatments — that we can no longer see the proverbial forest for the trees. Doctors have become like vultures, perched and waiting for diseases to appear, so that we can attack them with our arsenal of weapons, to the point where we totally ignore the possibility of preventing them in the first place, and thereby sparing the bearer much misery and pain.

The good news in all of this is that such a system already exists. Although it is not the current standard bill of fare, it is readily available to anyone who goes out looking for it. And the way to find it is simple.

First of all, you can become personally responsible for your own health by beginning to read some of the excellent books on the market on subjects such as nutrition, exercise and fitness, stress reduction, and general wellness. In addition, you can seek out one or more of the increasing number of physicians of all kinds who are starting to appreciate the wholistic approach to health care.

A very important step toward your personal goal of optimal health is to find yourself a good chiropractor with whom you are comfortable working. He or she will not only take care of the structural integrity of your body, but will pay careful attention to the other important health factors as well.

And certainly, you should have a medical doctor, but the one you ought to have may not be the one you have now. You should have one who is willing to work with you — and with your chiropractor — in a combined team effort with the ultimate objective of lifting you higher and higher on the health ladder.

A sensible approach would be to utilize the services of both professionals, and anyone to whom they may occasionally refer you, in an ongoing program of health maintenance. The job of both doctors should be:

(1) to maintain your good health by careful administration and application of wholistic health principles;

(2) to attend to any health problems that do arise; and,

(3) to educate you as much as possible about how to apply the principles of health to your particular lifestyle.

Your job is to *assume responsibility* for your health by following their recommendations and making conscious choices that support your well-being. If you handle your health in this manner, I can promise you entrance into a whole new arena of wellness that you probably never knew existed.

There is one more issue that needs to be addressed: the question of *incompetence.* As is the case in any occupation, some chiropractors are better than others. Some are more richly endowed in the areas of tact, human relations, clinical judgement, and technical ability.

In most fields, such individual differences are of relatively little importance, the only significance being that some people might earn more than others or climb the ladder of corporate success more quickly.

In health care, however it is quite a different story. The very health and lives of people are at stake. There is no room for incompetence. But ncompetence exists in health care, as it does everywhere. For that reason, it is mportant to choose *all* your doctors carefully, preferably on the basis of reliable referral. And, don't be afraid to *interview* doctors before making a choice, asking them questions about their background, training, and approach to the care of your health. The patients who have most impressed me have been those who followed this course.

Beyond the question of competence is another issue. It must be kept in mind that all doctors are human, and that even the very best are subject to human error. Doctors make mistakes. Health care is far from an exact science, and results are often unpredictable. There's much that we don't know about the body — in fact, what we *do* know pales by comparison. All any doctor can do n diagnosis and treatment is his or her very best.

What troubles me most of all in this area relates to the general image of Chiropractic. Specifically, it relates to the way in which people most often react o an unpleasant or unsatisfactory experience with a chiropractor.

When a person has a bad experience with a medical doctor, it's *the doctor* who is bad, or *the doctor* who made an error. However, when a person has a bad experience with a chiropractor, it becomes an indictment of *the entire profession*. The customary reaction to such an experience is along the lines of "Uncle Charlie was right — those people *are* quacks. I'll never try *that* again!" And then, the person goes out and propagates that kind of sentiment.

The point is this: it's important that you keep Chiropractic in the same perspective as Medicine, and that you apply the same standards to doctors of both disciplines, realizing that a single bad experience with one doesn't mean that the whole bunch are inferior. All a bad experience means is that it was a bad experience. Hopefully, now that you have some knowledge and understanding about Chiropractic, you can appreciate its value and will not be deterred from seeking its many benefits.

There is one last philosophical observation to be made. It has to do with the Life Force that pervades all of us.

Not only does it affect each of us individually, as the compelling force of life, but I feel strongly that the Life Force is part of what connects us as a race of beings. It is an Intelligence far beyond our cognitive ability to understand it or figure it out.

If that is so, then attempting to control it is clearly not the most sensible thing to do, and health care should not be an attempt to manipulate, alter, or deceive it. To me, it would seem that a system of health care that *facilitates the ability of this power to express itself* makes a great deal more sense.

A system, perhaps, like Chiropractic.

APPENDIX

North American Chiropractic Colleges

Canadian Memorial Chiropractic College: 1900 Bayview Avenue, Toronto, Ontario, Canada M4G 3E6 (416) 482-2340

Cleveland Chiropractic College: 6401 Rockhill, Kansas City, MO 64131 (816) 333-8230

Cleveland Chiropractic College: 590 N. Vermont Avenue, Los Angeles, CA 90004 (213) 660-6166

Life Chiropractic College: 1269 Barclay Circle, Marietta, GA 30060 (404) 424-0554

Life Chiropractic College - West: 2005 Via Barrett, San Lorenzo, CA 94580 (415) 276-9013

Logan College of Chiropractic: 1851 Schoettler Road, Chesterfield, MO 63006 (314) 227-2100

Los Angeles College of Chiropractic: P.O. Box 1166, Whittier, CA 90609 (213) 947-8755

National College of Chiropractic: 200 E. Roosevelt Road, Lombard, IL 60148 (312) 629-2000

New York Chiropractic College: P.O. Box 167, Glen Head, NY 11545 (516) 626-2700

Northwestern College of Chiropractic: 2501 West 84th Street, Bloomington, MN 55431 (612) 888-4777

Palmer College of Chiropractic: 1000 Brady Street, Davenport, IA 52803 (319) 326-9600

Palmer College of Chiropractic - West: 1095 Dunford Way, Sunnyvale, CA 94087 (408) 244-8907

Parker College of Chiropractic: 300 E. Irving Blvd., Irving, TX 75060 (214) 438-6932

Pasadena College of Chiropractic: 8420 Beverly Road, Pico Rivera, CA 90660 (213) 692-0331

Pennsylvania College of Straight Chiropractic: 7500 Germantown Avenue, Philadelphia, PA 19119 (215) 248-1100

Sherman College of Straight Chiropractic: P.O. Box 1452, Spartanburg, SC 29304 (803) 578-8770

Texas Chiropractic College: 5912 Spencer Hwy., Pasadena, TX 77505 (713) 487-1170

Western States Chiropractic College: 2900 N.E. 132nd Avenue, Portland, OR 97230 (503) 256-3180

INDEX

Also by Dr. Richard E. DeRoeck

TOTAL ALIVENESS: The Key to Effective Living. Impulse Publishing. Softcover, more than 160 pages. Publication scheduled for Fall, 1989. $14.95.

This remarkable book by the author of *THE CONFUSION ABOUT CHIROPRACTORS* can open an endless number of doors for you in life. Intended as a guide to living a fully effective and optimally functioning life, it can wake up the sleeping giant inside of you. Dr. DeRoeck breaks down what he calls "Total Aliveness" into four primary components, and gives you a formula for full self-expression through these four elements. Every area of life is covered, from health and well-being to control over your circumstances to making a real difference in life. This is a resource book for living the kind of life you've only *wished for* — the kind of life that you've thought only *other* people led.

Don't delay! Discover the keys to effective living. Dare to be all that you can be in life. Order *TOTAL ALIVENESS* today, so that you can receive it the minute it comes off the press.

ORDER FORM

Impulse Publishing
P.O. Box 3321-B
Danbury, CT 06813-3321

Please send me_____copy/copies of *THE CONFUSION ABOUT CHIROPRACTORS,* by Dr. Richard E. DeRoeck @ $9.95 each.

Please reserve_____copy/copies of *TOTAL ALIVENESS: The Key to Effective Living,* by Dr. Richard E. DeRoeck @ $14.95 each, and send it/them as soon as they are available.

I understand that I may return any book for a full refund if not completely satisfied.

Name _____

Address _____

_____ZIP_____

In Connecticut: Please add sales tax of $.75 *(CHIROPRAC-TORS)* and $1.12 *(ALIVENESS)* for each copy.

SHIPPING: $1.00 for the first book and $.50 for each additional book.

M)